UNDERNEATH THE FLESH

By Alexandra Gallagher Mearns

'One million people commit suicide every year'
The World Health Organisation

Published by:
Chipmunkapublishing
PO Box 6872
Brentwood
Essex
CM13 1ZT
United Kingdom

http://www.chipmunkapublishing.com

Proof-read by Elena Yiatros

ISBN: 987-1-84747-073-7

UNDERNEATH THE FLESH

**My life as a Morbid Obesity Sufferer
and a
Compulsive Overeater**

Alexandra Gallagher Mearns

ACKNOWLEDGEMENTS

This book is dedicated to:

my son, Edward-James and daughter, Abby-Rose; my late mother, Sandra Mearns Gallagher (Bulimia sufferer); my late father, Patrick Gallagher, who never got to know me as a daughter or a woman; my surgeon, Iain Macintyre, who gave me my physical life back when I was facing death head on; my dear friend, Julie Moffat, who has been my rock; my old pal and social worker, Gordon Clapton and finally Women onto Work (WOW) who believed in me and got me back onto the road to employment. And not forgetting those, who allowed me to cry, share and explore my pain, and listened to me and my world of food.

INTRODUCTION

My compulsive overeating / morbid obesity robbed me of 35 years of my life. It took me to psychiatric hospitals; it took me down roads of humiliation and life saving operations that only your worst nightmares take you to.

The world of isolation and judgment I have lived through with this compulsion, words cannot describe.

I have never experienced hunger or I have never experienced fullness. I have experienced being 28 stone and 11 stone.

I have experienced two periods of my life in intensive care. I do observe three 12" scars over my body by getting my flesh cut away on a daily basis, and this illness has left me permanently disabled.

I have experienced every method that is out there for weight loss from herbal remedies to obesity clinics.

I have experienced head and heart hunger.

All the time, people referred to me as FAT, but what FAT always meant for me, and always will, is feelings and thoughts. So I invite you to read about my very dark world, where I became an expert on one hand and very much in the dark on

the other hand.
This poem is my invitation to you.

My World of Food

Come with me to my world of food,
I will let you see how it alters my mood,
And gives me those desired feelings of feeling good,
The sugar highs and lows always topped up to make me feel high,
I am one step closer to that place in the sky,
Quickly shut down the feelings of fears,
And let no one close to see the buried tears,
As only I have understood this world, to you it may not yet be clear,
Because food has been my friend, my love, my enemy,
And I invite you to read of my 35 years.

UNDERNEATH THE FLESH

THE EARLY YEARS

I can always remember the first feeling of feeding the emptiness. It was with a packet of pink and white marshmallow sweets. I was 4½ years old and in my Grandmother's house. I just had to finish those sweets, and I can remember feeling physically sick (and I was), but I just had to finish them. (If I had realised the powerfulness that packet of sweets would have over me I would have binned them.) I just had to get to the sick/bloated-stoned feeling that would stay with me for the next 29 years.

I was the youngest out of my sister and myself. She was a year and four months older than me and we stayed with my mum (Sandra) in a block of new-built flats in the south side of Edinburgh. My mum and dad divorced when I was four and I firmly believe this was when the compulsion started.

My mum and dad had married in 1966 because my mum was pregnant. They were both 17 and my mum soon fell pregnant with me after my sister. Seemingly, my dad had an affair when my mum was pregnant with me and maybe this contributed to the distant relationship between my mother and me.

My mum and dad, when they were together, were always at each other, shouting or in silences. When my dad was around, the living room always seemed to be dominated by the sound of horseracing coming from the TV (one of my father's compulsions was gambling).

I had my dad on a pedestal. I loved him so much, and like most lassies, I was going to marry him when I grew up. Mum and dad had favourites, I was my dad's and my sister was my mum's.

Living in Holyrood Court (the flats) was OK. There really was not a family unit. We all stayed in the same house but it was like my mum and sister versus my dad and me. Quite a lot of the time my dad's brother, Frank, would stay with us. He was a small, thin man who always looked much more powerful when he was drunk and that was 80% of the time. There was always drink flying around the house, not on a daily basis, but at the weekends (Friday through to Sunday there were parties in the flat for the adults). We were packed off to bed around 7 to 8 o'clock and would drift into sleep listening to loud voices singing songs to "I left my heart in San Francisco" (Uncle's favourite song) with a high possibility of being woken with arguments or drunken brawls once the drink had hit the magic number.

I was very scared of drunken people. There was a lot of it around, in my home and on the estate where we lived. We constantly would travel through the Cowgate in Edinburgh, famously known for homeless people and alcoholics and I always held my mum's/dad's hand tighter when we walked through those streets.

Nothing was ever discussed with us about my dad leaving. I got up one morning and he was gone. After 4 or 5 days I came to realise that he was not at work and not coming back. I remember so vividly sitting in my bedroom, on my own, on my rocking horse and feeling so rejected, abandoned and alone. Self blame, what had I done so wrong that had made him leave, self-will came in, I would get him back. (Those feelings were very powerful and controlling in my relationships in my adult life.) The feelings of loss were so intense that is when one of my masks came in, pretending to my friends that my dad was working away, not wanting or being able to accept the separation. I was not allowed to mention my dad's name as whenever I did to my mum, I felt daggers of anger from her. She would make it clear by her eye contact and body language that we were not to talk about my dad. My sister and mum bonded closer together at this time, and if ever I have experienced intense periods of loneliness in my life, this was one of them. It was my sister and mum against me and I was angry with my dad for leaving me to deal with all this.

Food was definitely my main comforter at this period in my life. I was eating lots of flour based food and at school we got free school dinners, so there was always second helpings.

My home life with my mum, sister and my alcoholic uncle was just a base to stay. There was not a lot of happiness going around. My mum cared for me on a practical level, giving me food and keeping me well dressed. My mum had my sister and I like two dolls, up to her eyes in debt to stores/catalogues because we had to be the best dressed and it was all for the benefit of other people. Probably to keep things clean on the surface, so that no one could see we were falling apart on the inside. All my mum's friends were on low incomes as well but we always had to have the best. We had to have the best clothes, hair bone combed on a Sunday, and a spotless flat with 'mod-cons'. We were the first to get a colour TV, round about 1972, in the flats. Neighbours would come in and look at it and the pride in my mother's face that she had achieved this purchase. My mother was on Social Security but had a cleaning job in the morning as I always heard her boss being mentioned as, "A greedy, tight bastard".

My mother was a very, very attractive woman with long, red hair, all the latest fashionable clothes (she was only 22 or 23 years old) and she turned male heads. She knew she had this power and I felt jealous of the attention she got from men, also mixed with anger as I didn't want other men looking at my mother – that was my dad's place. I hated her and blamed her for him leaving.

I felt so, so alone with my mum and sister, I did not enjoy those days (isolation played a big, big part in my illness.) My mother was a great woman to be around, fun and playful, if she wasn't doing the 'sipping water days'. The 'sipping water days' were bulimia, but back in 1971/72 there was not a strong medical diagnosis of this illness I suspect. The 'sipping water days' could last from 3 to 21 days, and you always knew when those days were there because my mother would cut herself off, bury her head in a book and speak to us very, very angrily. She was agitated around preparing food for us, and I felt her anxiety, moods and distress strongly. I can remember one of the 'sipping water' episodes. When the electricity was cut off and my mother was sitting in front of the gas oven in the kitchen with her feet up at the door and a candle burning to help her read her book. She was so distant from us and in the candlelight looked so alone and unhappy. We played around the kitchen like little mice. Not much conversation, just the light of that candle and oven and feelings of emptiness. That candle/'water sipping' episode seemed to last forever. It is strange how time looks and feels in a five-year-old life.

Money was obviously tight at this time. The electricity was cut off and our new colour TV was gathering dust in the corner of the living room. My mother would never let anyone know what was going on in the house; her pride and self-will were a strong defence in her personality. She was a very proud woman. That is why my sister and I had to have the best clothes, the best toys, and the best, clean flat, at the cost of the electricity being cut off. I think my sister and I just came to accept the times when the electricity was cut off. It was acceptable for us and we also knew never to tell anyone, not that my mother had ever said this to us. But we just knew, call it instinct or vibes, but we kept shut lipped about what went on in the flat.

I actually felt quite scared when my mother went on a 'water sipping' episode because the food cupboards were kept with the basics, usually tins of soup, beans, rice pudding. Cakes and biscuits were not free flow, and to someone like me, who was in the prime of my illness, I would have to think of other ways to feed the compulsion. I did this very well. I would get leftovers from school dinners. I would get sweets and crisps in my school bag from other kids. I would save my play piece for night-time eating. I would go round my friends' at tea-time and usually get the odd sandwich or biscuit while they were eating. I came to be a great forward planner and a person whose thought pattern was distracted a lot of the time thinking about food (a common symptom/pattern in eating disorders).

So I can honestly say that my mother's 'water sipping' days were, for me, unhappy. (Maybe subconsciously we were bouncing off each other's eating disorder or making contributions to it.) My weight was still at this point pretty normal for a child of my age and when the weight did start to creep on, it was called puppy fat, and puppies are cute and loveable, so it was OK to be a puppy. A lot of my eating at this time took place on my own in secret (another symptom of the illness). I would join in at mealtimes but always knew or needed to have food tucked away in my schoolbag or room or to have access to food via friends' houses, saved pocket money, but I always got by.

My mother at this time was starting to see other men and this totally distressed me. These men would come into our flat and were not at all interested in my sister or me. They would force affections on my mother (kissing, cuddling), and my mother, like some proud cat who had got the cream, would play the game with them, pretending to be cool and casual, but made up to the nines with a short skirt on, heavy make-up, strong perfume and either ready for verbal attack or defeat. Most of these men, from what I remember, were unobtainable, either married or living with someone else. They always seemed to be strong, tall men that would protect my mother (but only for a short while). I hated those days and I hated my mother each time she met someone new, whether it be Bob the social worker with 2 kids of his own, or Fred the married man who ran a pub, or the policeman she chatted up after a drunken night out. She would always say to us that they would be our new dad and I hated her, wished her dead, for saying this. My own dad, at this point, was making spontaneous visits and at times being intimate and close to my mother. We would always get quizzed on my dad's visits about what mum was up to. I hated the power and time she took up, if my dad wasn't with her, he was talking about her. I felt jealous of my mother and could read her quite well as a child. My mother knew the power she had over me, but still remained unhappy. I had great problems at 5 years old, coping with people being affectionate to each other. My mother's brother, Andy, who stayed with us once, took me on an outing to the museum with his girlfriend and they were holding hands and kissing and I had this major tantrum. I threw away the stick of rock they had bought me and I cried. They were puzzled by my behaviour. I felt anger, jealous, left out and sheer sadness. (My mum and dad had probably been separated 6 months at this time.)

The impact and scars that were left on me after the divorce carried forward with me for most of my life. A lot of the time I opted to stay at my grandmother's house with her and my granddad. I didn't enjoy being at my mum's and I was a favourite of my grandmother's. My granny and granddad were typical Edinburgh southsiders, born and brought up there. They stayed in a ground floor tenement and had for the past 30 years. There was only one bedroom in my granny's flat and she had brought up 7 kids there. Her and my granddad would sleep in the living room on a push-down sofa bed, and I would sleep beside them.

I had a closer bond with my granny than anyone (mother's parents), but she always referred to my dad as a "bastard" and I didn't like it when she spoke like this. My granny was a plump, small woman with long, black hair and a jolly face. She walked with a limp (disability due to brain haemorrhage) and always wore a 'pinny' (apron). She smoked Capstan cigarettes like a trooper and loved a big tipple of rum and coke. She was a great provider of food. She had food contacts all over the place for someone who was semi-housebound. She knew everything and every food contact. There was Rab, the Ice-cream maker, over from her flat that, surprise, surprise, had a notion on my mother. My granny would send my sister or me over for big, huge Pyrex dishes of ice-cream, fresh, ready made (for free, of course). Then there was her brother who worked for Millar's sweet factory and got the odd bag of sweets (or 20 bags) and there was the Jewish bakers round the corner who would sell things very cheaply at the end of the day, and the last time that I can remember was being sent for a 1p bag of chipped fruit. So my comfort of going to my granny's was a compulsive overeaters paradise, anything from ice-cream to bags of cakes, fruit, etc. My granny was never out of her scullery (kitchen), either always cooking 'big, fat chips' as she called them and homemade batter for her fish.

My granny was a tough woman and took no-one's

shit. Her and granddad had a fiery relationship. They were either gossiping about someone or fighting verbally like cat and dog. My granny would have his tea on the table or at a low 'peep' (flame) in the oven. He would come in about 2:45 in the afternoon as the pub shut about this time. We would always get the sniff of stale beer in the hall and my granddad would talk a drunken talk, have his dinner, fall asleep in the chair and then get up every evening like an alarm for just before 6 o'clock and do the same pub routine over again until closing time at 10 o'clock.

My granny and granddad lived off social security, but now and again my granddad would do the odd job for someone 'on the side' as they called it (cash in hand). He was a joiner, but he only did this for his own beer money, or sometimes he would bring in people's TV's or radios that they had put out for the bin, do them up and sell them. My granny's hall was like a junkyard. I always got the impression from my granny that she was happy when my granddad was "out of the road" as she put it. She would refer to him as "a drunken, old bastard", and if he came home drunk she would go through his trouser pockets a lot and take the odd pound. (He got wise to this and started putting his money down his sock.)

My granny loved her rum and coke and every Friday night she would arrange a party as she called it for my sister and me. This same routine happened every Friday and usually started about

6 o'clock. The small coffee table was laid with free sweets, coke, bars of sugary tablet and crisps. My granny would put on the old blue record player and my sister and I would dance to Abba and Brotherhood of Man. My granny would clap us on and we had competitions for the best dancer, but there was method in my granny's Friday party nights. This was to get us so tired that we would be in bed by an early hour and hopefully sleep through, because Friday nights were my mum and granny's night out to the local pub. The plan was my mum, with her good looks, would get chatted up by various different men and both of them would get drinks bought for them. My sister and I were left in the house on our own and I was terrified.

Various different uncles (one being my granddad's brother, who was known as 'Ringo') would sometimes stagger into the house drunk. My sister tells me that he sexually abused her and I witnessed it and soiled the bed. On one of those Friday nights, my mother also found out, went 'haywire' and it was all hushed under the carpet (Ringo is dead now). I really can't recall much of this incident, but I do know that he would stagger in drunk on Friday nights, so Friday nights, for me as a 5 year old child, were mixed with fear and excitement – excited about the sweets/sugar hit and fear about being left on our own. Little did I know at this early stage that fear and excitement would play a big part in my compulsion.

The weekends were always full of drink. If it wasn't drink in my granny's house, it was drink and parties in my mum's flat. My compulsion was getting pretty obvious by now (age 6). My mum was getting irritated at me putting weight on. She would say how fat I was getting or how much cake I wasn't allowed to eat, always making a big sound in front of other people, making me feel shame and disgust at myself. My dad's visits at this stage were becoming fewer and fewer. There was a lot of anxiety in my life and lots of isolation and loneliness. Food was my only friend, enemy, comfort, drug.

Sometimes I wonder at this stage, sub-consciously if I was maybe setting myself up for what fate or distress lay in front of me – the death of my mother.

CHAPTER 2

THE DEATH

I will always remember the day that I was parted from my mother. It was just like any normal day, coming home from school, but as soon as I saw the ambulance at the bottom of our flats, I sensed something (that feeling in my stomach that something was not right). My fear was confirmed when the ambulance man got in the lift with us and said, "Flat 6". My sister and I giggled, but I felt fear, silence in the lift and us following the men in the black uniforms. When they got to our door, the panic set in. My Uncle Andy (my mother's brother) let them in and ushered us to the side. When I saw my mother, she was sitting in the wheelchair, holding her stomach, pale and drawn and obviously in a lot of pain, but she still managed to smile and comfort us and told us, "Not to worry, she would be back soon". She left with the ambulance men and my uncle dealt with us. We were to stay at my granny's until mum came home. We took our favourite dolls and walked the short walk to granny's house. I felt anxiety but I also knew I would be fed 'good-style'. Granny's was a stodgy house, pies, chips, cakes, sweets, etc. My sister was more distressed than me, but we stuck close together. While staying at granny's, we temporarily moved school after mum had been in hospital for 2 – 3 weeks.

My compulsion was getting all it required and major changes were going on, new home environment, new school, and no contact at all with dad (Granny wouldn't put up with "the bastard" as she called him). My sister and I visited mum every Friday, still dressed like her little china dolls. We wanted her to come home and kept asking, we were wearing granny out.

There was huge anxiety and worry around for everyone as the weeks turned into months. Mum went into hospital in August and we were well into October. The change I remember clearly is when mum got moved from the Infirmary to the Deaconess Hospital. She changed. She was moody. She was not her hopeful, happy self. (The Deaconess was a hospital, similar to a hospice, last place before death.) The strange thing was this hospital was the building right next door to my granny's home where my mother had spent all her childhood playing and here she learnt that she was going to die at the age of 26 from bowel cancer.

Things moved very quickly after she was put in that hospital. There were loads of adult silences, loads of getting sent out to play. Shut away from our mother's death. It was decided by the adults that my mum would go and stay at my Auntie Ann's (her sister) and my Uncle Billy's, who would care for her in her last days. This was October / November 1973.

I was pretty OK with being at my granny's house. I

could feel that something was being kept from us and we were not told how ill mum was. I was well into the food at this time and was getting my feelings and emotions fed with the food. My sister and I were saving up for a Christmas gift for my mum when she came home. Each week in the silver box, we would put two pence each away until we could get her a good present. The day we chose the present, we were going to visit her at the weekend. We wanted to get the best present we could. It was the end of November and we had saved up 50p. At this point, we had not seen my mum for 4 weeks (which is a long time for a 6 / 7 year old). The present we chose, after much squabbles and fights, was a Christmas plastic wreath with Santa and Rudolph in it, all silver tinsel and in clear cellophane. We also had change left over for a chocolate toffee apple each. My granny had bought us new clothes to go on the visit and we would dress like twins in our kilts and new tops and our hair in bunches. The trip to my Aunt's was three miles away, and a part of me looked forward to it. I had that fearful, anxious feeling in the pit of my stomach (which I seemed to be having a lot of these days), but I knew very well how to cure that – there were sweets or chocolates in my pocket like a little comfort blanket. When we arrived at my Aunt's, it was good to see her two daughters, Edith & Jane, but on greeting us, we were told to be quiet, no noise. We went into the living room and the coffee table had apple pies, sandwiches and biscuits. That coffee table gave me great warmth and reassurance that day, as I knew, even without exchange of words, that I would need it.

I was a bit scared to see my mum. She was bed-ridden in my cousin's room. The wait seemed like ages and the adult silences were frightening me. I really just wanted a food hit! My sister and I were finally allowed to go in to see my mum. Behind the door, my mum tried her hardest to smile. She frightened me. Here was my mum, the beautiful mum with the long red hair and voluptuous body, gaunt, pale, looking drunk (morphine), probably about 5 – 6 stone, looking death in the face and leaving her two wee dolls behind. She asked us to come over to the side of the bed. I felt fear and tiny in that room. I thought of the coffee table with the goodies. I obsessed about the coffee table. We gave my mum her present and she never even took it out of the cellophane, which puzzled me. My sister was physically closer to her. I was beside my sister. My mum's smile faded as she started to cry. She told us that she was going up beside the angels and we were to be good girls for her and she would always be a star in the sky watching over us. My sister was crying. I wanted to get out of the room and to fill my face with those apple pies and biscuits. I was confused about the gift – had we chosen the wrong one, is that why it was not getting opened? I didn't understand about angels, stars, death, but I wanted to get out of that room. My mum kissed us and I got released. My sister stayed for a few more minutes. I didn't want to be in there and could not cope with the emotion. I went back to the living room and the food was given the green light and boy did I scoff those apple pies and biscuits... If ever I needed a sugar hit / sedative effect, it was then. I didn't understand as we took the trip back to my granny's that night. Was that it, was that the last time I would ever see my mother? All I could think of was the present that she gave us to take back unopened, not being able to understand why she had rejected it and the feeling of disapproval that she didn't like it, failure of making the wrong choice. My sister was still upset and we had the bloody adult silence yet again from my granny and uncle.

My mum died on Saturday 8th December 1973. My granny and granddad did not have a telephone and I can't recall the time. It felt like lunch-time and my granny's brother (Wullie), our great-uncle, came in and I remember him saying the words, "I have put a red rose at her side." Then there was hysteria from my granny, colour drained from my granddad's face and the words from him, "No my lassie". My sister was crying her eyes out. All I felt was confused as if I was some sort of outsider looking in. I really didn't understand what was going on and felt the fear feeling in the pit of my stomach. I did not want all this confusion, isolation, and fear. Food played a big comfort that day.

The next few days went in a haze. Nobody physically sat my sister and me down and told us what had happened, the adult silences were intense and the grief raw. Drink was shielding the feelings for them and food for me. My weight at this point was no concern to the adults around me; all I had was the cute puppy fat, nothing too drastic yet!

Life was very different at school. Glances of sadness and sympathy came from teachers and silent whispers amongst them. In a way, as a 6 year old, you felt pretty noticed, here you were getting all this attention and totally confused why, because no-one ever sat me down and explained about the death of my mother. Maybe they could not comfort me if my emotion got too raw or maybe they just felt totally uncomfortable themselves, but looking back I really wish someone had given me the truth and respect I deserved. It was even decided by the silent adults that my sister and me should not attend the funeral of my mother, so we never even got to say goodbye on that final departure.

Food was free-flow now. I always remember the dinner-ladies feeding my sadness and grief and I knew how to play the part. I would willingly hang about the dinner-hall, offering to help clear up plates, dishes and even got to know most of their names. May was the one in charge and June was obviously someone who was an addict to the food game. She was a big woman. I felt needed in that dinner hall. It gave me great comfort in my life, as I needed it badly. Seconds of school puddings would come my way, without any problems. While all the other kids were playing or mixing with each other, I was one of the Dinner Ladies Crew. The feelings of comfort and isolation fed my compulsion and warmth from the providers. After lunch, play with kids didn't hold much fun for me. Dinner halls were much more my scene.

On the lead up to that Christmas, it must have been the bleakest time for all of us. I felt very much that we were left on our own at my granny's and granddad's. There was a house full of people always coming round with sad faces and expressing their grief. A lot of this would be done through alcohol. Of course, not forgetting us, we would be given sweets and packed off to play or into the room to play with our dolls.

I can't remember my sister and I talking much about my mother's death, probably because we had not been with her for 3 months, we did not realise fully that she was not coming back. I do remember my sister briefly mentioning my dad at this time, as far as I was concerned, I only had feelings of anger and betrayal for him.

Somewhere in those three weeks it was also decided, yet again by silent adults, that my sister and I should go and stay with my Aunt Ann and Uncle Billy, who had nursed my mum. I remember this being told to us very briefly in my granny's house.

Because my aunt had cared for my mum and my cousins did not have much for Christmas that year, we were to give them one of our huge selection boxes, filled with sweets. Can you imagine how this felt for a compulsive overeater? – Sheer and utter hate at the thought of having to part with my food-drugs. I felt more loss over that selection box in that period of time than anything else. I felt like crying, screaming, kicking and punching. This felt like the last straw having to part with some of my fix, because I now understand how the food compulsion catches on so quickly, it grips you like sinking sand. You forward-plan, your thoughts are very planned and calculated. You have powerful thoughts over the food and it has power over you. All this was being f****d up for me by the silent adults. I suppose it's like when an adult keeps drinking to hit or numb the same feelings I have. That is what that selection box was for me and it was all getting f****d up and f*****g my thoughts up. I took an instant dislike to my cousins at this stage.

Christmas of 1973 was spent at my granny's and granddad's. There were not a lot of cheerful, happy faces going about. My sister and I still got the excited feelings of what Santa was going to bring us and my granny and granddad did their best, the rest of the family helped out with money. Deep in my heart I think I still thought that my mum was coming back. Surely if she was not here for Christmas, she would come back for my birthday…But I had lots to occupy my mind, new presents and lots of goodies, sweets, biscuits and all the rich, sugar and 'stodge' that surrounds Christmas, so life was not too bad.

I can't remember any gifts from my dad that Christmas, but I still had feelings of anger and betrayal inside me and I would deal with him when I saw him. Little did I know that would be sooner than I thought!

CHAPTER 3

DEATH NUMBER 2 AND THE MONSTER

I can't remember when we arrived at my aunt's and uncle's to stay. I am pretty positive it was just after my 7th birthday, early January. The same old Madera cake and stale shortbread was used for the celebration of my birthday. It was always forgotten – no plans, no birthday cake, no presents, just a drunken happy birthday, song from adults around me, some bits of cash and Madera cake. I always had great resentment towards my mother and sister. This was because my sister got huge parties with pink cakes and lots of friends. Her birthday was in September.

My arrival at my aunt and uncle's house presented huge changes like school. Once again I had the feeling of fear and excitement on my first day at my new school. I remember having lots of sweets in my pocket to get me through that morning. At this stage, I still had no real concept of where my mother was. I suppose I magically thought that she was coming back (just like my dad), which played a big part in what I thought. This was approximately a month after my mother's death. I just did not cope well at all at the new school that morning, no matter how many sweets I had packed down my throat that morning. I was just not coping well. I had a big emotional trauma in front of the class. No matter how much sugar I had in my pocket, it was not giving me the comfort I needed. My aunty just stood there apologising to the new teacher. I just had lots of fear and worry about going into this new situation that once again, had not been explained to me by the silent adults. All this change was catching up with me at a funny rate and the food was getting packed in more than ever. Also the puppy fat was getting more like a round puppy, but there was never any mention of this from the silent adults, my food and me were left well alone.

I can't really remember too many outstanding dramas at my aunt's. We were kept clean and warm, given the comfort of a home and left very much to our own devices. Round about February, my dad appeared on the scene for little visits. It had seemed like an eternity since I had seen him. We were not warned about any of these visits. There was no way I was going to show him any sort of affection. He had betrayed me and let me down before, so I was not going to let him in again. On these visits we got showered with sweets and told that we were dad's little girls. Never once was my mother mentioned. My dad saw us once or twice before the final break of silence came. My sister and I hadn't seen him for 2 – 3 weeks and once again I thought he had gone away forever. I felt dreadfully sad and just ate a lot to get me through the unpredictable comings and goings of my dad. Then we were presented with the big question – did we want to go and live with him forever? There was no big in-depth conversation, just a big decision for a 7 and

8 year old to make. I was very clear in my mind that I didn't want to, but my sister was definitely going and I was definitely staying at my aunt's. The reason I was staying was because my dad was never going to be able to let me down or reject me or abandon me like he had before. I hadn't forgiven him and my gut feeling told me not to go (if only I trusted it). The guilt I was torn with was that my sister and I were going to be parted and I did love my sister. She was my playmate. I did not like the thought of being separated from her. I can always remember that torn turmoil feeling, I just didn't like it. A suitcase was packed for me just in case, when my dad arrived on that dreaded Saturday morning, I might want to go – big decisions for the small 7-year-old girl. I remember that sleepless night, my pride would not allow me to go, the guilt I felt about being separated from my sister and the fear I felt at being left behind. All this was going through my 'wee' mind and I could just not approach the silent adults.

The Saturday morning arrived. My sister was excited about seeing my dad. The room was oozing with her buzz. I felt the strong pride and anger that I would never forgive my dad – no way! I also felt annoyed at my sister for not being strong and wanting to go with my dad. Had she forgotten how he had let us down, walked out of our life before, and she was going to run to him with open arms. (Later in life she told me the reason she left was because my aunt's husband who we were staying with had sexually touched her.) When my dad did arrive, I stayed hidden in the bedroom. I could hear and feel the tension of the conversation between him, my aunt and uncle. They were civil, but only just! My sister was clinging to him like some pathetic rag-doll. They asked me if I wanted to go. I looked at my dad. He bent down and all my anger, pride and pain melted away. I ran into his arms like I had always envisaged. My hero, my long lost dad, being held in his arms made everything OK. The warmth and comfort I felt, words could not explain. We were all setting off on the new road of freedom. We were getting away from the pain of death, away from silent adults, away on a big, happy, new adventure (if only I had trusted that gut feeling in my stomach). We said our goodbyes, pretty quickly and promised to go back and visit. We had our suitcases and had to get two buses to my dad's new house. It seemed to take forever and we sat upstairs on the bus, as my dad wanted a fag. My dad's affections were wearing off now and we were starting to irritate him. I had this horrible feeling in the pit of my stomach and tried to ignore it. When we got off the bus at Easter Road, we walked down the grey street to stair number 5 where we would become victims of physical and mental torture…our prison at number 5. When we got there, my dad had forgotten to mention on our journey that he had a new wife, Tricia. She was sitting on the sofa and the flat was a room and kitchen with shades of dull browns and an empty, cold feeling. As soon as I met Tricia, I knew that I was jealous of her and she didn't like me. Here I was, I had just got my dad back and lost him to another woman. A guard went up. My sister played her usual role of people pleasing, 'yes', 'no' and false politeness. I was much more reserved and guarded. Food was coming into my head more and more. I remember that there were sweets for us that day, and for some strange reason I remember trying to make a cake for this Tricia as some sort of acceptance, approval, peace offering, with sliced peaches on it! I was pretty confused by all this change and a big part of me wanted to go back to my aunt's with my suitcase.

I suppose that day a part of my little girl dream was shattered. It meant that I had lost a part of my dad to another woman. I instantly felt when I met Tricia that there was an unspoken barrier of resentment between us. I will also never forget those drab brown colours of that flat that were to be a prison of sheer hell and misery for the next 7 years. I suppose we must have settled in quite quickly. The next thing that was presented to us was that we had a brother, Tricia's and my dad's son, Patrick. He was not there on the first day, but he appeared a day or two later. There was no communication, no warning, he just appeared. He was about a year old. My dad soon got back into the routine of going to the pub, of which the hours were 11 – 3. Tricia was to care for us. She also had another child, Margaret, who stayed with Tricia's mother. At this stage my head was totally screwed up. The food was passing my lips like some sort of fuel. I was at this stage, going over the puppy fat and just getting fat. So many changes had happened in 6 months, my mother's death, 3 house moves, a ready made family and another change of schools. We went back to the old school that we went to with my mum. I can remember that during the first few weeks my dad would pick us up like some Cheshire cat that had got the cream, like he had won, he had got his daughters. He would pick us up at 3.00 p.m. and try to look like the loving, caring father, but he was stinking of fresh booze and just a sheer embarrassment. This was not the dad I desired or knew or fantasised about. This was a stranger. As much as I felt the loss of my mother, I also felt the loss of my father. A lot of confusion was going on. I always remember holding his hand in public view but when the show was over, he would withhold his hands back into his pockets. Sometimes, if my dad had won on the horses (he was a compulsive gambler as well as an alcoholic) we would get sweets on the walk home. After a few weeks, my dad's tendency to pick us up from school wore off (his compulsions were more important), so we would walk home ourselves. I can always remember the first time ever really crying for my mum after her death. I had been staying at my dad's for about 4 weeks and he and Tricia were out for the night. Tricia's sister, Aileen, was babysitting us and this was my first meeting with this woman. I remember just bursting out in tears. She asked me why I was crying and I explained that I wanted my mother. This woman hammered me, battered me across the head and about the face. This plump, overweight woman had battered a small 7-year-old girl that she had never met before for grieving for her mother. I then got sent to my bed. I felt terrible and I was told when my dad came back that I was going to get battered for being cheeky! The next morning, after a fabricated story, my dad hammered me and told me I was a cheeky little bastard. My sister watched with silent, sad eyes. This was to be the first of many beatings that would come my way! So I had just the feeling of being left with the death of my mum and the death of a dad (I had fantasised of a loving, warm, kind dad). All I was left with was an angry, evil monster. My dignity, pride and self-esteem were getting drained away, all the stuff I thought that had been built into me in the first 6 years with my mum. Manners, clean clothes, warm comfort, good hygiene were all taken away in a matter of months. Things were slipping fast and furiously. My dad was drinking daily. Tricia was struggling, the flat was filthy and my sister and I were barely getting by. We slept in a small box room, as it was only a one bedroom flat. No window in it, a double bed, no wardrobe, just blue bags supplied by Edinburgh Council for rubbish to keep our clothes in, no drawers. Toys were limited. The flat was freezing and had no bath or shower, just a toilet. There was no toilet paper, just newspaper to wipe ourselves with, no toothbrushes – so very drastically, the little china dolls that belonged to my mum, her pride and joy, were becoming little tramps (that was to be our new title at school). It was pretty obvious that my dad and Tricia didn't want us there. It was my dad's pride, getting back at my mum's family for not being accepted and my mum divorcing him, that he obviously never got over, which made him want us. This anger and pride had led him to want us, not for fatherly love or compassion towards the grief of the death of my mother. I was struggling with feeling angry with my mother for leaving us, not being there to take practical care of us. I was living in a place I didn't want to be. My dad was a monster of anger and Tricia was resentful and angry at having to share 2 kids with her man. My emotions were numbed sadness, grief, loneliness, anger, fear – all had to take second place...this was the survival game now. Food would get me through this. I was now an addict to food. I had ways and learned great manipulation skills that would get me my daily fix of food. For all that had been done to me by these dysfunctional adults, I still had that child innocence of sincerity in me and wanted to be loved and liked. I knew that I was only a 7-year-old girl but inside I felt about 20 years old. I knew when the 2 deaths had happened that my childhood was over. I wanted to be big and strong to be able to stand up to the battering and neglect. I came to learn to show no emotion to it. I pretended that it wasn't going on. To the outside world, I wanted to put on the show that everything was OK, that no alcohol or beatings were happening, I had to hold it together and I was, in my eyes, with food topping me up. I was getting fatter by the day and my appearance was letting me down, my clothes were shabby. I was stinking of urine due to bedwetting and I was protecting the crazy adults. My role in the family was the strong one. I would wait at the hall or front door like some scared, cowering puppy on the inside waiting for the monster that would come in about 3.30 p.m. I always went through the same ritual in my head. Would he be in a good mood? Would he be in a bad mood? The feelings of anxiety and fear would never leave my stomach. I would question… what did I do so wrong? Why did he hate me? Why did he batter me? I actually felt like some masculine man. I did not feel like a 7 / 8 year old girl. I would stare him in the face and take the beatings on the head, the slaps, punches and kicks. My dignity and pride would not allow me to cry because if I cried I had given in, he had won, I would have been defeated. My sister was always the victim, who would cry very quickly, but the more I stood up to him, the more he gave. I suppose everything has to have an end result and I thought his was to get me to cry, no way, the pride I held on the exterior was award winning, but inside I was crying – crying with fear, despair, shame and hopelessness. If the monster couldn't be bothered to batter my sister or me, he would get us to fight each other over at the far end of the living room. He would set us up, like two fighting bulldogs. We expressed sheer sadness to each other before one of these matches started, but we knew we had to amuse the audience. We would kick the shit out of each other and he would shout, "Come on fatty, boot her" or "Come on Mo" (as he called my sister) "grab her hair, get her down". I think I would have rather had the beating from him as he knew how close my sister and I were and he just wanted to break any bond that we had. The sister-to-sister fights were the worst times, because afterwards we would cry, say sorry to each other and comfort each other, and I would escape to food. You may wonder if we were so poverty stricken, where food came from. Food came from the kind old woman that was the manageress of the bakers called McAnish. Each day after school, I would go in, they shut at 5.00 p.m. and Mary, who walked with a limp, just like my granny and wore the same type of apron as my granny, gave me the comfort I needed to get through the days of hell and distress. I never once had to utter any words but I knew she knew what was going on. She may have seen the pain in my eyes or my dirty appearance, and she was feeding me and caring for me. I did love Mary. The goodies that were on offer were vanilla slices, cream buns, pies, sausage rolls, milk-loaf bread, hot cross buns and strawberry tarts in the summer. There was unlimited food. Mary would give me one or two carrier bags of food, and before I got back to that flat every day at 4 o'clock, I would have at least 4 or 5 cakes, pies, bridies and boy did I need this, it fuelled me up for the night ahead and to deal with the drunken monster. It suppressed my fear and gave me courage to face them. I also had May in the shop called Smiths that sold loose biscuits by the pound and they had broken ones that they could not sell. So guess who got them? Also Smiths sold sliced cooked meat and sometimes May would throw in some ends of ham or beef. If I didn't fall back on Smiths, I had Jan or Jean in the fruit shop who would give me fruit and then I had Marie in the newsagents at the bottom of the stairs. In return, on most days these people would get me to go to the butchers, dry cleaners, do their shopping, etc. I would be repaid with cakes, biscuits, mostly 5p or 10p daily from Marie or Jan or Jean. This was used towards my sister's and my sweet money during the school week or saved at the weekend. I had a little system going and the two crazy dysfunctional adults that were abusing and neglecting us knew nothing about it. If they did, it would have been taken off us for drink. The leftover bakery goods we would hand over, but not the cash. I was definitely the caretaker of my sister. Anxiety and fear just ripped out of her and I always got us by. I did things that I was forced to do and stripped me of any dignity I had for myself, but at that stage I was beyond that feeling of caring.

CHAPTER 4

BABYSITTERS / THIEVES

Tricia was the total opposite of my mother. She wore no make-up, was not very feminine and was certainly not house-proud. Ever since day one, I could tell I was going to have great conflict with Tricia. She liked my sister a little bit more than me, but my sister was like a little lapdog around her. Tricia used to give me some beatings and what I always remember about the beatings from her were despite the dire poverty we were living in, she had about 9 rings on her battering hand and one of those was a full coin sovereign ring and God did I feel the impact of that ring on my head. Tricia gave mean blows. She didn't miss for all of her small frame. She was like some kind of female lightweight boxer. Every day I got a beating from Tricia. I was always reminded that when the monster came home, she would tell him and it was round two from him. Tricia could not cope, she did not do weekly shopping or clean the house, there were no sheets on the beds and the smell of stale urine was in the flat from me wetting the bed or my brother Patrick's towel nappies lying soiled. Every day Tricia would go to her mother's with Patrick who stayed in the Cowgate and she would leave my sister and me in the house. We had to light (or get ready) the coal fire, wash dishes, and sweep uncarpeted floors. We were not allowed to go up to Tricia's mother's house and if we ever did have to go with her, we would have to wait in a swing park. From 10 in the morning to 2 in the afternoon in the rain, snow, any weather, but in the early days we got the joyful tasks of cleaning the flat. This suited me as I could go to the bakers, fruit shop and get food and money. My sister would make a deal that she would do the housework and I would provide cash and food. I felt like some sort of man going out to work to provide basic essentials for my sister and I, but that was our routine. Tricia would always be back for 3 o'clock as the monster would roll in then and she would have to get his tea ready. He would come in, physically or mentally batter us, then have a sleep until 5 o'clock and she would wake him up for his tea. He would only eat things like steak and chips or chops. He would snort and splutter like some sort of pig. He would get his tea served to him. A few times he threw it at Tricia with the words, "What the f*** is this". He also would have a special spicy sauce that we would have to fetch for him. His conversation used to be about what horse had let him down, how he was going to work in Germany or about some p***head in the pub (he was actually a bricklayer). We would get something like the pies from the bakery or smashed packet potato and spam. We would eat separately from my dad. Tricia would always buy Patrick sweets and leave my sister and me out. This really hurt me, so off with my saved secret money; I would buy my sister and me sweets that we could eat at our leisure. My dad would go back out most nights. He would go out about 7 o'clock and come back at 10 o'clock.

Tricia would just watch TV and smoke and we were sent to bed about 7.30 in a freezing, cold box room without a window, stinking of stale piss. School, at this point, was just a refuge. No enjoyment was coming out of it or playing with other kids, it just became a place to get away from the craziness of what we had become exposed to. I can always remember teachers' faces looking at us with pity and sadness. They could see our appearance going downhill rapidly and all we got were silent, sad looks. The bruises from the beatings were hidden a lot, either on our arms or legs, covered pretty well. Dad and Tricia could have got an award for their covered-up punches. All the time I saw the sad, silent teachers, I wanted them to rescue me. I did not want to expose my dad or Tricia (strange how kids who are being abused will always have some sort of loyalty to their abuser/s…)

Tricia did not drink very much when we arrived at the flat but most Saturdays she had decided to go out with my dad to various clubs. We were left with various different babysitters. One of them was my cousin who was 15 (Frankie). On one of his babysitting nights, he wanted to sleep in bed beside us. We were all in a double bed in the brown, smelly box room. He was at the back, my sister in the middle, me at the front. I was told to face the front and they were making noises and movements. The feelings I had then I knew were uncomfortable and wrong with regards to what they were doing, but I also felt envious of my sister getting attention, even though I knew it was wrong. I also felt he had rejected me because I was fat. I also felt shame and dirty at the uncomfortable noises my sister was making. I wanted to turn round and comfort her but I knew what my role was – to face the front and not turn around as much as my sister was being abused – so was I in the mind.

This cousin made it plainly clear that this was a secret and it was not to be told to anyone. I can't ever remember him coming back, but Saturday nights were always a dread in case we were exposed to any more abusers. If we were not exposed to it by direct contact, we would witness it by various adults who came back to the flat and would sleep on the living room floor with cushions and have sex. There was no door on the box room, just a ripped curtain that had many holes in it, so we could see what was going on or be woken up by sex noises (I have to say I was never directly sexually abused. I observed the abuse done to my sister).

My dad's drinking was getting totally out of control. Now I would be about 9 years old and as much as his drinking got out of control, so did my food, it was like a competition. I was my sister's caretaker and my dad's. I got the worst beatings because my pride and strength would not allow me to cry. Tricia, at this point, had another son, Anthony. Patrick was about 2 or 3 when she had him. My dad seemed to drink more and got pretty aggressive towards her. She would get the odd beating here and there and would always take it out on me. When I was about 8 or 9 years old, my dad informed my sister and me that we were too old to kiss him goodnight. This came as a mixture of feelings and thoughts to me. I felt relief that the angry, let down part of me didn't have to kiss that b*****d anymore, but I also felt strong rejection from the last straws of affection that were totally gone. At this point, I felt as if I had been in this mess for years, but it was only two years, the despair and hopelessness I felt was still there, but the strong mask had to still keep up the pretence that everything was OK. The denial was easier to deal with. I was probably about 8 stone now, which was pretty big for a 9 year old. I stuck out like a sore thumb. Grief for my mother had totally gone and it was just a distant memory. My dad allowed us no contact with my mum's family, but in my lunch hour my fearful stomach would lead me up to my granny's for a visit of 15 minutes. My sister would never come with me. One of my friends from school called Diane would 'chum' me. We planned the route through the park, over the hills, the back way, so no one would see us. The walk took about 15 minutes each way and my granny was so upset and relieved to see me. The anger she expressed to that b*****d would ring in my ears. She would always give us food, ice cream, biscuits and cakes. Seldom did I see my granddad; he was in the pub most days. I would visit once a week or fortnight. The fear in the pit of my stomach would not allow me any more visits. I was terrified of any adults that knew my dad and Tricia seeing me and reporting back. The visits would come to an abrupt end as Tricia got a job in my school as a cleaner. She would start at 6.30 in the morning and finish at 8.30, and then go back for 3 o'clock, which suited my dad's pub hours. She had taken various jobs that fitted around him and the pub. She had a part-time job in a bakery at Tollcross where we would live off pies, sausage-rolls and bridies for our tea – my dad still getting steak. One day Tricia had a huge fight with him in the bakery and by God we got beaten up by him in the street. He could not contain his anger. He booted us with those big wedged shoes on and a few members of the public asked him to stop. He told them to "F**k off" and "mind their own business". He lost the plot. We went to stay with his sister for 2 or 3 days until him and Tricia made up and it was back to the good, old dysfunctional system. When Tricia was working in the school, free dinners for my sister and I came to an abrupt end. Round about this time, I was checked by the dental nurse and she picked up that I had an abscess and had to be sent home. This was one of the worst beatings I got for telling the nurse and for letting the school check my mouth.

Any professionals that came into contact with us, we had fear of because we knew we had to hide the abuse. On one occasion, on Boxing Day, when I was about 8 or 9 and had my party dress on which was a long dress with the seventies wedger shoes, I was sent for a bottle of lemonade (glass bottle) for my step-mum's sister, who was another babysitter. We were to stay overnight as my dad and Tricia were away at their own little party in some club at Danderhall. I got the lemonade out of the chip shop at the bottom of the stairs and I was also to collect two empty potato sacks for the Christmas rubbish to go in. So balancing the sacks under my arm and the juice in my hand, I climbed about 3 stairs, tripped over my long dress and fell on top of the glass bottle face first. The glass caught my cheek and chin and I screamed. I was more scared of all the blood than anything else and about messing up my new party dress. A neighbour from the stair helped me up, and I could see the annoyance and fear in Tricia's sister's face about this inconvenient emergency. The ambulance men were on strike that year and no taxies were around with it being the festive period, so we walked to the Royal Infirmary, with me supporting the left-hand side of my face with a towel. I can always remember the weight and feeling heavy but that was not my main concern. It was getting battered for spoiling my dad's and Tricia's night out. I felt the fear of them coming to hospital. When we got to the Infirmary, we were informed that they could not take me as then they treated only those over 13 years old. As I was only a child, I had to go to the Sick Children's. They gave us an ambulance. My face got stitched up and I still had a fear of my dad and Tricia appearing. The doctors and nurses were kind. They gave me 35 stitches on my face and 2 in my gum.

By the time my dad and Tricia got there, it was about 11 at night, all false professional smiles and stinking of stale booze. I knew how to play the game – smile and make everything look happy; don't let anyone see the fear and anxiety. My stomach was already preparing for its protection from anxiety.

The doctors gave me a little bag of sweets, chocolate Santa's and festive things but it was a bit silly as when I got home I was nil by mouth for the next 24 hours and Tricia's sister's kids got my sweets. That was painful, handing my fix over.

I had a big, huge plaster on my face and a bandage. My dad or Tricia didn't hammer me that night. I just was the centre of attention with other kids, and then sent to bed. My face hurt and I was starving for food and comfort. My dad or Tricia never even asked how I was.

The next day Tricia was out with my sister, Patrick, Anthony and me and we were in the street and she slapped me across the face where the scar was. I felt hot and numb from the slap and I knew she wanted it to have maximum effect, and it did. It was painful but no tears, no crying, it was the pact to myself.

When I went back to school, I was in the spotlight for a week or two. I had to attend hospital and my dad had made a new name for me – instead of 'fatty' or 'Sandra' that he would normally call me it was now 'Cut Chin'. It always reminded me of some sort of wicked pirate name from the Captain Pugwash cartoon I would watch. In the house, everyone referred to me as "ask Cut Chin", "Where's Cut Chin". I suppose this was to be one of the kinder names than what the future held for me.

CHAPTER 5

COMFORT PEOPLE AND NAMES

Tricia's father was a kind person in my childhood. He was an English man that always wore a bunnet and would never go out of the house. He was quiet and a lot of the time you did not notice him around. He was an on-the-tap babysitter for Tricia and her sister. There was about six or eight children he would baby-sit.

Tricia's mother would never be out of the bingo. She was a hard woman with an aggressive reputation and the father was in the reverse role. He would keep the house, do the cooking, and baby-sit.

The house was always in chaos, never tidy. If not cluttered with material objects, it was cluttered with human beings. On the times that my sister and I were allowed in that house (which was not often as we were outcasts, even the other kids treated us like that), Tricia's dad was OK to be around. At night he would drink a few cans of McEwan's Export and he would be fine. Very rarely did I hear him shout, never swear, he just did not seem to fit in with the craziness. On one occasion he did snap and it was the words and expressions that he showed that made me see him as a decent human being. Tricia was beating my sister and me in front of him and he stepped in on this occasion. It was like he snapped. He hit her with disgust in himself only to make her stop and shouted, "They are not your kids to hit. Leave them alone! Why are you doing this?" It got the result he wanted. It made her stop and she cried, but I could see the disgust and let down in his face, all in those few minutes. Why did she have all this anger? Why had he resorted to feeding into hitting her? Feelings of guilt and shame came from him. I saw him as some sort of hero, some sort of protector, but I could always feel the gentle side of him. He just did not seem to fit into that family at all. He was taken very quickly and severely. One day my sister and I were out playing in the street where our flat was. It was a summer's day and Tricia's sister's son came down to tell my sister and me that we were to go with him. I could feel the anxiety (it's all I seemed to live off). When we got up to the home, adult tears, silence and grief was all over the house. Tricia's dad had fallen and hurt his head and died from the injuries. I could not stand the tears and grief. I went to the living room and laughed with a step-cousin. We were lucky, one of the adults knew it was a reaction to death and we never got hammered.

That was the end of my hero and protector. All I lived off, with faces of self-pity, were the people in the bakers shop, biscuit shop and all the people that I ran errands for. Teachers were the worst pity-givers, with their silence and inability to rock the boat and voice the abuse. I was probably about 10 or 11 years old now and about 10 stone, no longer a puppy, a diet of sugar and flour handouts given from people who cared through food! I was a mess. I could not even hold it together anymore. During this time, another guilt-ridden avenue I was forced to go down for food, compulsion and survival was stealing. Not just little things, out of shops, like sweets, but bigger things from an old lady neighbour who was going senile. I would go and do her shopping and take extra money or take 10p out of her purse. I felt dreadful and ashamed but my main purpose was to feed my compulsion and my sister – it was survival, but I hated what the B*****ds were turning me into. One time I stole £10 from a launderette money jar. I was full of fear and excitement. My sister and I had plenty of food that week and friends. I really did, at this point, hate what I had become, a disgusting mess, physically, mentally and emotionally. The self-loathing I had for myself was bad and the hatred from my dad and Tricia was just as bad. I did not feel like a child. Childhood has been long gone. I just felt lost in a world of food, beatings, stealing, fear, anger and let down. Through the times in the flat, my sister and I tried hard to stick by one another but a lot of the time I got sent to Coventry. Tricia would not speak to me for weeks or months. She hated me. She would speak through my sister or dad. I was just 'a nobody' to her. It sort of suited me because I disliked her intensely. At this stage, my nicknames were "The Blob" (because I was so fat), 'Fatty' or 'Cut Chin' (because of the scar on my face). Living with this on a daily basis within that flat made the aggression in me bubble, but I never showed it to my dad or Tricia. They even made my sister and Tricia's kids call me the names.

I hated not having a bath and I hated my body, which was now totally out of control at this stage. Every now and again I would get put on a *Ryvita* diet. My dad, through his drunken haze, would say "Look Blob, you're disgusting" and tell Tricia to get me on a diet, but all they could offer was *Ryvita* and stupid, crazy food that they thought would solve my compulsion. All I did was stuff my face with more bakery goods and secret eating was rife.

I remember one Easter, I must have been about 11 or 12 years old, and I got sent to bed for 2 weeks without much to eat. I was not to speak to anyone; no one was to speak to me. I was in a room with torn wallpaper, limited light, surrounded by blue council rubbish bags and stinking of stale piss. I felt at my lowest point then, unable to get food, unable to get out. I remember someone had given me a bible and I read it to the best of my ability. It was the only thing that gave me comfort. I felt like a prisoner. I know that incident was Tricia's making. I had said something and looked at her the wrong way and she sent me to that cell for 2 weeks. It is the worst I ever felt in that flat, laying still, seeing what my life had come to at the ripe old age of 11!

It would be a good time to mention that my dad

and Tricia were Catholics. My dad did not go to Chapel but Tricia did. Most Sundays she would go to Mass and Confession and come home and neglect and abuse my sister and me. All the rest of her family would call me a 'Proddie' (slang for Protestant). My sister had been baptised a Catholic as my mum and dad were together. I had not been christened or baptised, but I went to a Protestant school.

I remember looking around that flat and looking at holy pictures and asking God why I was being punished for being alive. Tricia made it plainly clear that she hated my mum, and my sister and I were just constant reminders of my mum and dad's life before her time with him. I heard her slag my mum off to her other sisters and during arguments between her and my dad. In the early days, all was referred back to my mum; my sister and I were only with them to fuel my dad's drinking and her cigarettes, and eventually her drinking.

Family allowance days were always a Tuesday and Giro days a Thursday or Friday. I got fearful of those days, as I knew the drink would be rife and I would get it.

CHAPTER 6

ABUSERS AND FREEDOM

High School was a nightmare. Because we were living in the pits of poverty and dysfunction, our appearance and body odour was bad. My sister was at High School before me and I started at roundabout 11 or 12. I made one or two friends. I was quite an aggressive child to my peers, I had to be for my protection, and so the friendships I formed were made on my aggressive strength, not on a give and take basis. I was not a bully, but had just been moulded into some protected, guarded, aggressive image. I had totally lost myself in the last 5 years. My hopes and dreams as a child were put on hold and I always wanted to be grown up to cope with the hell I was living in.

My dad's abuse and drink was in the pits now and Tricia was just a couple of steps behind him. My sister and I still had the strong bond, her, the victim and me the strength. Most weekends were spent around alcohol for my dad and Tricia. They would pack us off to Tricia's brother who lived in the West of Edinburgh in high-rise flats and lived with a woman who he had 3 or 4 kids too. They would baby-sit us at weekends and the fear and anxiety we had going there was dreadful. Tricia's brother was sexually abusing my sister and when she told me this I felt powerless, angry, fearful and anxious, because I could not protect her or save her. The build-up on that bus journey gave me a great fear knowing that my sister was going to be put through this. On one occasion when we went there, my sister and I arrived to find him in on his own. He had sent his partner to the chip shop that was a 15-minute walk away. On arrival, he told me to go over and get extra chips for us and I could see the cold fear on my sister's face. She knew what awaited her. I felt vast amounts of guilt, vast amounts of anger, but I had promised her that I would never let him know that I knew about the abuse. My sister's face was white. I waited for the lift but went back to the door, wanting to barge in…But like most abusers, he was making sure the coast was clear and made sure that I was getting in the lift. The fear and let down, the shame and guilt I felt in the pit of my stomach was immense. What had we done so wrong to be going through this? My legs ran all the way to the chip shop, as fast as my fat body would allow. When I got there, I could sense that his partner knew something was not right, but nothing was said. I hated my drunken b*****d of a dad at this point. I wanted to kill him for everything he was putting us through. My sister was badly abused that night and others that followed. We would sleep in the living-room and he was a bar tender and came in at one or two in the morning, wake up my sister, and take her through the kitchen that was just off the living-room, and make her touch him. My sister was so distressed and so was I. I can always remember my sister saying to me that he always made her feel sorry for him. He used to speak about his dad dying and about this being their secret. I heard the abuse and I witnessed it, the nights of him taking her out of bed, the aftermath of emotion, and the build-up of fear to Saturday nights. He knew that I knew because eye contact can say everything and I would stare at him with pity and disgust, and he knew that I knew. I hated men at this point. I really hated them. On one other occasion with my dad's real brother, I would have been about 13 at the time; they had all been out drinking. We were stuck in that smelly box-room, my dad pissed and Tricia pissed through in the other room. We were subjected to his brother, our uncle, lying masturbating, shouting my sister to go through to him. She was shaking with fear. He only shouted my name a couple of times. I can always hear that drunken repetitive name shouting. I told him to "F**k off". Anger overtook me. I had to take charge of the situation and put my fear aside. My sister shaking, him playing with himself, drunken b*****ds lying in their bed. I got up, walked past the animal, shouted I was going to my dad. His dick was quickly put away. I punched my dad's arm and told him he was keeping us awake. All I got from him was a drunken mumble, but it was enough to put fear into the drunken b*****d in the living room. Situation sorted. I slept that night like most with one eye open in case of the weirdo in the living room waking up, and also protecting my sister.

For some strange reason, all those sexual abusers didn't come or approach me. At the time I thought it was because I was fat and unattractive, but looking back, I think it was that they could see the victim in my sister and they could see the strength in me. I was probably too much of a risk to abuse because I may have opened the lid on them.

The beatings for me were dreadful and I was always not being spoken to. My final battering from Tricia came one summer's day. I had gone swimming with her daughter and I didn't get back until late. She battered me stupid. She was really hitting me over the head and punching me. I can always remember that she had long hair and I just grabbed it. I wasn't 8 or 9 years old anymore. I was 13. I gave as good as I got, as I was getting and she shit herself. I felt disgusted that this was what my life had come to, fighting back, lowering myself to their level. Tricia told my dad about it and I got hammered from him. I only lasted another few weeks in that house then. The worst beating I got before I left was from my dad. My sister and I had taken part in a sponsored charity walk and raised about £6. One night my dad was drying out and looking for money and I had hidden it on top of the wardrobe. He wanted the cash to go out for a drink. I would not tell him where it was and he battered me. He threw me against the door of the living room, and then threw me into the hall. I was just scrambling to get on my feet when my dad opened the living room door. I was lying on the hall floor and he kicked me full force in the face and slammed the door shut. Blood gushed from my nose. I was scared and when I opened the living room door, so were they. Fear and panic was all over their faces, the blood was everywhere. How were they going to cover this one up? I actually felt powerful for a few split seconds to see fear and panic and their faces. Dirty dishtowels and anything to stop the bleeding, which was not stopping, was put over my nose. They were both in a state of panic and probably scared that they would have to take me to hospital.

Eventually they got the bleeding to stop. My dad told me to get my coat on and he was taking me for sweets. At the ripe old age of 12 or 13, my dad wanted to take me for sweets. All my life I had wanted my dad to take me for sweets and I knew now was not about a kind act. It was out of fear and guilt on his part. Sweets were not going to make amends to me; a sorry might have done something, but yet again another f*****g silent long walk to the sweet shop.

Once we got there, I realised that there was stale bits of blood around my nose and a bump had formed (which I still have). The old man in the sweet shop knew me and knew my dad never brought me into his shop. He could see the pain in my face and I could see the pity in his. (I hated pity. I was crying out for adult action, but silence and sad looks was all I got.)

I never chose any sweets. My dad eventually

chose something. He was irritated at this point. I got the little white bag of mixed sweets, but it gave me no comfort.

Once again we walked back to that flat in an anxiety paced silence. We got to the flat, and then my dad went for his fix to the pub. I went through to bed and there whispers from my sister asking if I was OK. As usual, I had not cried, and had no intention to, but I knew I could take no more. I had lost my self as a person; my food compulsion was keeping me alive, but slowly killing me. I had to take action and I knew that my spirit was at its lowest point. Something had to change.

CHAPTER 7

CARE

A few mornings after getting my nose broken, my dad and Tricia were lying in the living room on a pull-down sofa. I was in my first year of high school. I had seen a bottle of tablets at the top of the cupboard. I was frightened but I could not exist like this anymore. I put the tablets in the carrier bag that had my schoolbooks in and called in for my friend, Yvonne. We walked along London Road to school, and I took the tablets in front of her. She panicked and so did I. She got me to school and my guidance teacher got an ambulance and I went to hospital to get my stomach pumped out. It was a horrible, frightening experience, and I was put on the psychiatric assessment ward.

My dad and Tricia were informed and notified that I would be seeing a psychiatrist the next day. They never came up that day to see me and I got a fresh, clean bed and a good night's sleep.

The next morning I saw a psychiatrist with a beard and told him that I was not going back to them or I would attempt to kill myself again. He asked me assessment questions and I went back to bed. I never said anything about what was going on in the flat.

I was waiting for them to come up. I was scared

that I would have to go back to them and get battered for exposing them. When they came up to the ward, they both walked past me and gave me a huge, filthy look. They went in together and spoke to the psychiatrist. They more or less said I was a nutcase; a wayward teenager and I had no reason to overdose.

It was decided that I was to go and stay with my dad's brother for a few weeks and a social worker would be allocated to me. I was happy enough not to be going back with them and they spoke briefly to me stating that I was a f*****g nutcase and that I was lucky my dad didn't take me home and batter me.

I stayed in hospital for another night and got things I hadn't experienced for years, clean sheets, a bath, proper cooked food, and I felt relieved that I was not going home to them.

I went to stay with my dad's brother and his wife, Ann, for almost a month. They had a son the same age as me. My Aunt was kind to me. At this stage I got a social worker called Roz and people came to speak to me from Welfare / Child Protection asking me what was going on at home. They seemingly interviewed my sister as well. The hospital had seen some bruising from previous beatings and teachers were now starting to put reports in.

At this stage I was a size 16 and probably about

12 stone. I was 13 years old and food was my crutch. I was using food just like my dad was using alcohol. Who knows, maybe if I never had the food, I might not have survived the years with my dad and Tricia.

It was decided, with my input, that I would go back and stay with my mum's sister, my Auntie Ann and Uncle Billy who had cared for me just after my mum's death. I continued at my secondary school and saw my sister briefly. She had been warned not to talk to me and fear was written all over her face. I felt so guilty for leaving her behind and I missed her.

On arriving at my aunt and uncle's, everybody wanted to put everything right and this was done by giving me nice clothes, a bath or shower daily, my first toothbrush since I left their home, use of a hairdryer (which I really didn't know how to use), etc. I never spoke about the abuse or battering. It was like everyone was tiptoeing around me, showering me with material and practical things, but the needle was in and the damage done.

My two cousins, Edith and Jane, who I stayed with, were put out by me being there. They liked it at first, but then started to get annoyed and frustrated with me (they were 2 years older than me). My social skills were nil. I didn't know how to hold a knife or fork or sit at a table. I always cleared my plate first and had no manners or civility. I had lost myself as a person and was buried under the food.

It was at one stage decided that I should go on a diet. The thought of this killed me. I started to hide food and hoard it away. I was asked to clear the table and I stole a bit of ginger cake and nearly got caught, so I hid it down my cleavage and could feel it getting moist and sticky, and I went to the bathroom and ate it.

I went to the local high school while I stayed at my aunt and uncle's and every day I would buy a packet of orange or custard creams and carry them in my pocket like some little toddler with a comfort blanket. My peers didn't accept me that well. I got called 'fatty' and 'fat slob', but I was grateful because the names of smelly and tramp were gone and I was starting to become semi-acceptable to society (but not to myself).

It didn't last long at my aunt and uncle's. I couldn't cope and still had to sabotage any form of care that came my way. It was decided after a few runaway attempts that I went back to my dad and Tricia's.

Once again it was a failure, and they basked in it, failing. They sat with each other and confirmed that they were right; I was just a nutcase (maybe I was). I lasted about 3 weeks back there. I was never intending to stay. Tricia gave my dad a choice one Sunday evening, it was her or me. My dad told me to get out. I was terrified, but I never showed it. It was about 6.30 at night, semi-light, and I walked and walked and walked. I was about 13½. About 3 in the morning, the Police spotted me and asked me what I was doing. I said I was waiting for a taxi for my dad as he was at a party. They knew I was lying. They took me to the car and took my details. I was frightened. I told them the truth, "Dad had thrown me out". One of them said, "We are going down to fill him in". I didn't care. They asked me where I wanted to go. I said to my granny's (my mother's mum). Off they took me. (I do believe they did go down and visit my dad, as they were angry that he had put a minor out onto the streets. My sister informed me.)

My granny and granddad gave me the basic, practical and homely things I required, but all my granny said about my dad was that she f*****g hated the b*****d. I started to become the carer of my granny and granddad. My granny was disabled and my granddad had TB. The food was rife, fish suppers, pies, cakes, and chocolates. I didn't want or need to steal to get food because it was on tap. Once again, I was Sandra, the carer (I had just got out of being a parent to my dad). My life, once again, was put on hold, tending to everyone else's needs…But it wasn't that bad as I had my crutch and didn't have to worry about where it was coming from.

My granny and granddad would drink at night, argue, and then go to sleep. My granddad got hospitalised at one stage for his TB, and we all thought he wouldn't pull through, but he did.

I didn't last long at my granny's, maybe about 8 months. I was tired and down and not getting the care I needed. I sunk further into despair and food. I was about 14 and 14 stone. My school friends were all wearing fashionable clothes. I was wearing what could fit me. They were all talking about boys – who would want me! …The 'blob' – 'cut chin' – 'fatty' (so I just kept saying I hate boys).

I was fed-up of my granny talking about my mum. I wished my mum were here. One day I sat in my room and cut myself and cut all my hair off. I hated what I had become. My uncle took me to the doctor who referred me to a Child Psychologist who told me that I was Endogenously Depressed (meaning from the past, not reactive). I was given amitriptyline anti-depressants and told to attend weekly, and if my situation didn't get any better, I would have to come in as an in-patient. After a few weeks it was decided that I was to go in. I went into a residential psychiatric unit for children with various different problems. Once again I was put on a diet and given 8 different types of anti-depressants each day (with the side effect of making you want to eat). I was not coping well without my crutch and needed my food but it was not so easy to get when it was being observed and controlled by nurses and dieticians. I was on a 1,000 calorie a day diet, and I was not coping with the loss of food, the sugar highs and lows, and with all the medication getting pumped into me, I started to get aggressive. I could not express what I needed because I thought that the main thing I needed got taken away from me, food.

My dad was phoning the patient phone drunk and giving me mixed messages that he wanted me to go home, but on the other hand, how I had ruined his life and aggressive talk. He frightened me more by these phone calls, still battering me mentally.

At one stage, I got very aggressive, and was disgusted that I went to the level of violence that had been inflicted on me – I hit a nurse. I got put to bed for a week with a major tranquiliser (Lagartel) that is used to sedate people with major psychiatric violent tendencies or outbursts. This was given to me and my food was taken away. My head and feelings were hungry but once again the professionals wanted to tackle the exterior.

There was one other girl in the unit with an eating disorder, anorexia. She frightened me with her appearance, and I must have frightened her with mine, but in a strange way, we became friends. (We must have known we were sufferers of eating disorders and had symptoms at different ends of the scale.) I didn't last much longer there, it was decided after another major outburst from me that they could not keep me there for the safety of patients and nurses. So once again, I returned home. Once again there were more beatings, once again mentally abused.

I lasted about 3 weeks and then got in touch with my social worker and said I had had enough. I was always frightened of going into care as I had heard horror stories and I did not want to go to a Children's Home.

My social worker informed me that my dad would need to sign me into care. I sat in the car at the bottom of the stairs and a part of me always had this fantasy in my head that my dad would come down, put his arms around me, say sorry and everything would be OK. The social worker came back with the signature.

The 15-mile journey to the Children's Home outside Edinburgh seemed like forever. I arrived there and got allocated a Key Worker called Jack. There were teenagers there of all different ages, ranging from 12 – 16 years. My stomach was churning with fear. I saw the other residents looking at me and making their judgements. I was badly overweight and only wore clothes that could fit, nothing fashionable, and nothing trendy. They all wore jeans and the latest fashions, so once again I was different.

I was taken to my room and introduced to the rules and the kitchen. Jessie, the cook, cooked meals that children liked and there were always snacks on the table. I took a lot of food up to my room and hid it for night time eating.

The Children's Home cared for me practically and gave me nice clothes and pocket money. No diets were forced upon me but my weight was always spoken about, either at staff meetings or with my Key Worker. I think I had a crush on my Key Worker. I never spoke to him about the past, but he was just a sort of person who I grew to like (not trust) in my time in the Children's Home. One guy, another resident, who was 15 years old, tried to come on to me. He was my friend's boyfriend and one night I was glue sniffing with him and two other people (glue-sniffing was the 'in-thing' in the Children's Home and I tried it about 4 or 5 times along with smoking fags). He tried to kiss me and touch my breasts. I didn't even realise that I was going into womanhood. I had started my periods. With no help or input from other people they had started on a stay at my dad's and I just coped. I rejected the boy's advances as I was confused and my mind was confused. I started to get frightened of him. I started to run away from the Children's Home.

Also, another female resident there was a friend of mine and the gardener of the Children's Home was sexually abusing her. He was a dirty, skinny, old man that smoked and had a hut where he kept his tools and he would take her in there. One day I went in and he was doing a sexual act. He knew I knew and I could sense he felt threatened by me. The girl involved asked me not to say anything.

I may have had good practical care in the Children's Home but I wanted out. I could not cope, so I just ran away, took another overdose, ate more food and was classified out of control. It was decided at a staff meeting that I should go to a locked secure unit. Two emergency social workers were called and took me to the locked unit where I made some good mates. I was OK in a locked unit. I didn't have to face the outside world, food was on tap and each day was a daily routine. I stayed there for about 6 months and it was decided now that I was nearly 16 and nearly legally an adult, so I could go into a care hostel for adults to learn independent living.

Once again, another move, a pattern there; I only stayed for 6 months. I moved into the social work unit and took a good couple of months to settle in. The food there was a luxury. There was a cook called Mrs. Higgins who was from the old school. She would cook everything from scratch and it was stodgy food, such as chicken pies, millionaire's shortcake, home-made jaffa cakes, etc. The food was on tap and a bulk of weight went on, while I was there, very quickly. I didn't have to hide food there as I had free access to it. My weight was pretty much accepted in the hostel by the staff and residents. There were only about 8 residents and a barrage of staff.

The staff were very liberal and politically minded. They took us on political marches and exploited the social work resources for their gain, getting trips paid to France for holidays, not much of our choice, but theirs. They ordered the best of food and did their own laundry in what was meant to be our home.

One member of staff brought me in home-grown grass for my 18th birthday as a gift. I smoked this and had a bad reaction to it. I got paranoid. I thought I was dying. I started going to the doctor's with panic attacks. I was a mess. My weight was about 16 stone. I was having panic attacks and I was on the dole.

I found a job, which paid cash in hand in a chip shop (a compulsive overeater's dream). I worked there 6 nights a week; I ate chips and fried food from 4.30 p.m. – 12.30 a.m. with the odd sweet or tub of ice cream. In the 7 months I lasted there, my weight was now about 18½ stone. I left there as it was close to my dad and Tricia's house and they kept pestering me for loans of money from my wages. I saw my sister once or twice a week. She had a job in a supermarket and was involved with a man who was a friend of my dad's; he was 10 years older than her, and God he gave her some beatings (a few times she ended up in the head injuries ward). She ended up marrying him.

My living accommodation was coming to an end with the social work. I was just over 18 and they were closing the hostel down. They wanted to rid of the staff to various different units, as they were

too powerful teamed together with their political views and their outspoken ways. They exploited us to gain whatever cause they wanted to get noticed, but we were young and naïve. It was decided, with the help of my Field Social Worker, that I would go into a shared flat with another girl. All the things that the hostel was meant to teach me for outdoor life, they never did, budgeting skills, cooking, washing, it was all done for us…
But I had survival tools inside me from my past.

I was frightened of the change that was in front of me and once again I took another overdose. This seemed to be a cycle – fear, overdose, and stomach pump. Back to where I was going. There was never any counselling or talk about how I had got to care or about what I was feeling. There was a file held on me, probably about what judgements or assumptions professionals had come to, but never once had anyone said to me or took me aside and asked me how I was feeling. One thing I did know was that I felt lost, f****d up and I was a great actor. One good thing that did come out of the hostel was that a member of staff put me in touch with a counselling organisation that would help me look at some of my demons.

CHAPTER 8

BACK TO SOCIETY

When I left the hostel, I got a flat with a girl of 19, whom I had met through the hostel. At this stage, I had started going to counselling and met a therapist who dealt in Art Therapy. She was an ex-Art teacher, old and kind.

At this point in my life I was totally unacceptable to society and me. I wore size 22 clothes and permanently looked at the ground. I had my hair covering my eyes so that I did not have to maintain eye contact with anyone and I felt a lot of shame and guilt. I had lost myself as a person and was buried under food. Every now and again, when I got a glimpse of myself in a shop window, I denied to myself that it was me. It was someone I had become but who was the 'blob,' 'cut-chin-scar-face'.

Jessie May, the therapist I saw for about a year, on and off, spoke with me about my mum's death and my life with my mum. I opened the lid briefly about my dad, and then shut it, as it was too scary. We never spoke about my need to eat or what I was feeling, we always tiptoed around this.

One of the good things that had come out of my life in social work care is that I made one true friend called Julie. She came from an alcoholic home and understood me. We never spoke about our childhood much when we were in care but we had a bond, a bond that sometimes does not need words to connect.

My life in the flat was strange. The girl I shared with was having problems with her sexuality and wasn't sure what partner she wanted to be with, male or female. I didn't even think of boys or men. I was 18½, other people around me spoke of s*******g guys and feeling them. I was curious but not that interested.

My sister had gone on to marry the clone of my dad. Every week she would be in hospital with a battering. On a few occasions I went back to my dad and Tricia's to visit. It was like a magnet, I couldn't keep away. They still 'slagged' me off and degraded me. Every time I went, I had to give them cash or baby-sit. They went on to have 2 more sons, who were 1 and 2½.

The house was disgusting. They had got a dog that kept having litters of pups. The pups would s***e and p**s all over the flat and the dog would eat it. Tricia and my dad were drinking badly. The two young boys were left with anyone and p****d on the lino floor so much without it getting cleaned up, that it leaked down to the woman in the flat underneath, who couldn't understand how Tricia's washing machine was leaking in the middle of the floor. Thankfully, for some of their young years, the two youngest got put in to day care in a social work nursery. If social workers were to benefit my dad and Tricia, they would be used. Obviously, there was some sort of file on the family now, and I got battered for bringing them to the door, but obviously they 'cottoned on' to how to use the system.

I was not coping in the flat with money skills and my black spells. I had no job, as I felt unemployable. I had no grades from school. I just felt what I felt every day, a big hole, a big void.

At this stage, I met the first person I would sleep with and, surprise, surprise; he was a clone of my dad, he had jet-black hair and was living in a social work hostel for recovering alcoholics. He was 5 years older than me and called Norrie. There were no dates, no great romance. Probably, he connected with my compulsion and thought, let's go for it. I knew how to behave and react around him; I could handle alcoholics because I had 10 years experience. We had sex and I kept my underskirt on. I only did it to see what all the talk was about. I wasn't really in the room and after it I thought, is that it! Norrie dumped me the next day. No problem to me, another rejection – another binge on food. I would spend my days eating, sleeping, and taking care of my granny and granddad.

The flat thing didn't work out and I moved in with my sister and her husband who were running a chain of dodgy bed-sits and getting housing benefit. My sister was putting on a show of how happy she was. She had nice, new clothes, soap, toothpaste, make-up, a hairdryer and a husband that battered her almost daily.

I got very little support or follow-up care after coming out of social work care. I was just put into a flat and left alone. I had always dreamed of being reunited with my sister. I didn't bargain that each night I would hear her getting battered. I could not cope with this and I was eating more and staying in bed. I was just back to my childhood and I could not rescue my sister.

I f*****g hated men. Why did they have so much aggression towards women? Here I was, back in a situation, listening to my sister's cries and getting battered for just being alive. A few times I confronted the evil little d**k but he just got aggressive with me. He never hit me, but threatened it.

I lasted about 3 months in that flat / bed-sit and ended up walking the streets one night, seriously going to kill myself. I ended up phoning the Samaritans from a phone box. They persuaded me to phone my doctor. My doctor told me to get a taxi to the local psychiatric hospital where a duty psychiatrist would see me. Half of me wanted to go, half of me didn't want to go, but what else did I have.

Breakdown Number One

When I got to the hospital, I saw the duty psychiatrist who asked me a series of questions and suggested that I come into an admission ward for a break. I was having bad panic attacks and a dreadful fear of dying before I went to sleep every night. I would shake all over and be convinced that I was going to die.

In the hospital I was put in an admission ward where people around me had very serious mental problems, manic-depressives and schizophrenics. I was being observed and watched to see what unit I was to go to. It was decided that I was to go to Ward 1, which had a 4 – 6 week waiting list, but dealt with group therapy and was a specialised unit.

I was so frightened in Ward 6, but I could still get food. There was no restriction on it, and there were 3 meals a day and a hospital shop so I could get my night-time stash. A few times in Ward 6, all my past thoughts and memories came back to flood me and I got angry and aggressive. A few staff nurses had to restrain me and I would be sedated. I just couldn't express myself, my head was f****d. It was a scary place, maybe all the years they had said I was a nutcase, I was one, and this is where I would spend my adult life.

A couple of social workers from the hostel where I stayed came to visit. They felt guilty about me being there and showered me with gifts and sweets. My friend Julie came up a lot and always encouraged me to stick in and keep fighting the battle. My Aunt and Uncle, who had taken me in when I was 14, also came to visit, but I still couldn't express myself. All these people were rallying round with support, but I had my support food, my loyal old friend and comfort.

On one occasion, a psychotic patient attacked me as he was hearing voices and having delusions about me. He physically hurt me and once again I wondered if I deserved to get battered and attacked.

After about 6 weeks, I went down to Ward 1. Dr. Cox ran this unit and there was a mixture of people; bulimics, anorexics, post-natal depressives. Each morning we would get up and have breakfast, then have an hour of group therapy. Until then my weight had not been mentioned. In one of these meetings, we started to talk about overweight people and my view was that I was disgusting (I would never look in a full-length mirror). Dr. Cox replied that some people found overweight people attractive, like African people. This didn't mean that much for me.

It was at this stage that it was decided in my care plan that I would be put on a DIET. One member of staff would shadow me everywhere and sit with me until I finished my meals. I was also on about 3 anti-depressants a day (side effect wanting to eat) and tranquilisers when required. The withdrawal period from sugar and flour was dreadful. I shook, I cried, I felt empty, I could not concentrate, I could not get my hands on food as I was followed everywhere by a nurse. Why were they doing this to me? Why were they punishing me? My comfort and crutch was taken away. I withdrew deeply into myself. I sat at mealtimes like a kid until I ate good old diet food. Sometimes I threw it in the f*****g air or at the nurse. I felt so humiliated like a bad child, being watched and told what to eat. These meal times could last from 15 minutes to 2 hours.

A lot of the food was new to me and I didn't like most of it, but I would be made to eat it. Eggs and fish are not foods I like and most of the time this is what came prepared from the dietician. I just felt so low and empty. I had come to hospital to get help and here I was getting punished for being FAT.

This plan lasted for about 6 weeks and it was not working, so the next step was to get me on weekend pass stays, and this was to happen at my aunt and uncle's. Also, someone from the supported accommodation social work team was going to come and set up a place for me in the community.

Word had got back to my dad that I was in hospital

and one day he came to visit, semi-sober, still stinking of the drink from the night before. I spilled my heart out to my dad, all about the sexual abuse of my sister that was f*****g my head, like some rewind videotape, and all the rest of the things that happened. He seemed concerned and told me he would sort it. At one point he smiled at me like he did when I was 4 years old and I thought, right my dad will sort this, everything will be taken care of. All he did was go down to his local pub, played the poor victim, got everybody to buy him a drink, and phoned my sister, who was told to get her a**e up to the pub. She went with her husband and in front of everyone; my dad asked my sister if Tricia's brother had sexually abused her. She denied it and Tricia and my dad went on to get drunk and confirm to each other that I was just a head case and in the right place.

My sister told me Tricia's brother got to hear about it, strongly denied it and it was just brushed over as if they were talking about the weather. Once again, my dad had betrayed me and rejected me.

At this stage my food was no longer getting monitored, and it was decided that they would treat the depression and once I came off anti-depressants, I alone could deal with my weight at weight watchers. I was beyond weight watchers. I was 19 years old and 19 stone, but I was happy enough just to get my fix.

I was in hospital for about 7 months and supported

accommodation was set up for me in a house within a Family Unit until I could be found a shared flat. I shared a room with a girl and the woman who ran the house was called Mrs. Cormack who was very overweight, so was her husband. They had a big house and took in foster kids and foreign students for extra cash. Mrs. Cormack always baked or cooked loads of food, so my compulsion was taken care of. I was very lonely, as there was nothing to do during the day. I started to walk around shops and started stealing small things that I didn't need.

I had not been back to my dad's since coming out of hospital and felt a magnet drawing me back. I didn't feel I belonged anywhere. One day I stole money from my room-mate and went down to visit my dad and Tricia. I was taking a big gamble as the last time I had seen him was when I was in hospital and had exposed Tricia's brother. I knew I could not go empty-handed, so I went down and bought their affection – I gave them a 'tenner'. Nothing was said about the talk in the hospital and they went to the pub. I was left to baby-sit each day. I would go down and visit them – I was back in. When I went back to where I was staying, the girl I shared the room with was so upset about me stealing her money. She did not blame me or accuse me. She was so distressed and I stood and lied and pretended to help. She eventually left the accommodation quite quickly after her money went missing...But what did I care, I needed it more than her, and I was back in with my family!

Moves and Battering

Eventually the social work department found me a shared flat with other people that had been in care, 5 minutes away from my dad and Tricia. Four other residents shared it and it was through a local housing association. My life was a daily routine of compulsively eating, going to the shops and walking around and stealing, getting things on credit that I could not afford and running up huge debts.

I would go down to my dad and Tricia's about 3 times a week to baby-sit. They still referred to me as 'fatty' or 'the blob' and spoke about me constantly. One night my dad and Tricia were out and I was baby-sitting. They came home drunk and my dad started on me. He slapped me, I stood up and gave him one f*****g punch, even I was shocked and said, "I am not 7 now!" He staggered off to his bed.

My dad would constantly appear at my flat drunk at all hours when Tricia threw him out. At first, I let him sleep on the couch, and then my flatmates got fed up with it. So my dad would just knock on the door until he fell asleep on the landing. Even at the ripe old age of 20, I was still not free.

My stealing was horrific. It went hand in hand with

my eating. My attitude was that I hated the world; it had failed me and owed me. One person who became friendly with me from hospital invited me to her house. She had an eating and drinking problem. On leaving, I stole her cashline card and stole cash out of it. The police came and charged me. I pled guilty and got a fine and compensation was awarded. I didn't care. I had a great food binge with the money and treated my dad and Tricia. My life of crime didn't stop there. Tricia's daughter had a boyfriend who broke into people's houses and stole their chequebooks and cards and I went out and defrauded them. I was so frightened not to say no, I wanted to be a part of a family at any cost, and I got great praise from my dad and Tricia. They got the goodies and I got very little, just enough to feed my compulsion and shut my mouth. One time my dad even came to six off-licences with me but wouldn't come in, but he carried the booze and fags. I felt appreciated and wanted. I went on to get a further two charges of fraud and very narrowly escaped prison – I got community service.

I was still having major panic attacks and was always going to my doctor. I was back on anti-depressants and a regular at my doctor's surgery.

I was now 21 and my weight was staying around 19 – 20 stone. I was not going around with people my own age. I just existed.

The Housing Association told us quite sharply that

we had to vacate the flat. I had nowhere to go. My friend Julie from the hostel had got back in touch with me. We got a flat two minutes away from my dad and Tricia. I actually felt pretty secure being near them. We stayed in this flat for about 5 months, during this time we went camping in Spain, which was a nightmare for me as I would not wear summer type clothes and stayed in most of the time. I stuck out like a sore thumb. It was a dreadful holiday. Once again my weight and compulsion deprived me.

On coming home, there was a big fight with me, my step-sister, Julie and Tricia's family, all about stolen goods. The police were involved and Tricia got charged. Tricia's daughter attacked Julie and me, and brought cousins and aunts all to back her up. Julie's family also got involved; it was like a gang war. My dad sat in the pub and drank, nothing to do with him, his words.

At this point I decided I wanted out, I had f*****g had it. The council offered me a flat on an estate 5 miles away from my dad and I took it. It was a tower block and I was on the 3rd floor. I got it ship-shape with help from a DSS grant. I decided at the age of 21 I wanted to do something with my life. I started to diet and lost a bit of weight and got accepted for a hairdressing college course. I felt pretty good for the first time in a long time. Things were OK.

I started going to weight watchers and counting

calories. I started having a social life with people from college. One day I was pulled aside by two of my tutors and told I was in the beauty industry and I **had** to go on a diet (I had lost about 2 stone in 8 weeks). I felt deflated, I felt s***e, I was being humiliated once again and not accepted. It was pretty tough being the biggest person in the class and being around people of acceptable weight. The tutors made me feel like the minority and I felt myself slipping back into the isolation and the food. When I put 4lbs on one week, I was called bad and naughty at weight watchers. Here I was, fast approaching 22, and I was bad and naughty and humiliated in a room full of people seeking the perfect solution to their weight problem. Needless to say, I never went back. I also continued to hate the tutors who had 'slagged' me off about my weight.

I hadn't seen my dad or Tricia for about 4 months and started going out with my friend, Julie, at the weekends. It was at this point I met Ritchie.

CHAPTER 9

LOSS AND BETRAYAL

Ritchie was 10 years older than me with dark hair and a scar on his face. He looked quite aggressive and he drank and smoked hash. Ritchie took to me right away and I clung on like some lost teddy. I was attracted to the age difference, nothing else.

From the night I met Ritchie, I had that feeling of fear and excitement in the pit of my stomach, but bit-by-bit, he started to unfold his past. He was in prison for 5 years and found coming out to society scary. Perfect! I would mother him and he could father me. He took me home to meet his mum (who was Catholic). He had just lost his father and Ritchie had to deal with this in prison. He also had an ex-girlfriend in Blackpool who he had taken drugs with, held up a shop at knife-point and got 5 years. I didn't care if he was a mass murderer, as long as he cared for me. Two weeks after we met, he moved in with me. He decorated my flat and cared for me. Two months after we met I felt strange, my breasts were sore and my period was late. I was pregnant. Ritchie seemed ecstatic, so did his mum and sisters. It was November 1988. We decided to get married. Everything was going so fast and for once in my life I went off food due to pregnancy sickness.

I was organising the wedding cake through the college and flowers and we were going to get married in January 1989. My whole life was changing, but I could cope. We went to meet my dad, in a pub of course, and for some strange reason we decided not to tell him I was pregnant. We met my dad in the centre of town. My dad shook Ritchie's hand and as he had no money we supplied him with drink all night. He said he would be at the wedding. Even when Ritchie went to the toilet, there were no good lucks or are you doing the right thing, it was the uncomfortable silence.

About 8 weeks into my pregnancy, towards the end of November, Ritchie had arranged to go and see his mum and meet me back at the flat. I got there at 3 o'clock and at 3.30 I had a sinking feeling in my stomach. I phoned his mum and she said he left her house at 1.00, so he should have been back at 6 o'clock. I went to check in my wardrobe. The wedding rings were gone and a ring I had bought for my dad's Christmas present. I knew the feeling in my stomach from the very start was right. I had been used and stolen from and all I could feel was anger and stupidity. All that kept going through my head was my dad, Tricia and her children laughing at me and saying what a stupid fat blob. I knew I would get no comfort from them.

I phoned Ritchie's mum and she said that she had given Ritchie the £1,000 his dad had left him in his will and presumed (or knew) he was away to Blackpool to be with his ex-girlfriend. I felt ripped apart and fully consumed by anger, nothing else.

I put the practical wheels in motion. I left college; I collected the cake and flowers and pretended to my friends that we were delaying the wedding. I went to see my doctor and arranged for a termination. I was so lost and in a lot of denial. I was back to the comfort of overeating. I told my dad the wedding was postponed due to Ritchie getting a job down south. Ritchie's mum stopped answering the phone to me. I wrote to her and told her what I thought of her.

My termination was booked in for 9th December 1988. The night before I had my overnight bag packed like a shambles, the way my life had become as always. I would pick myself up and get on with it. The 8th of December was the anniversary of my mother's death. She had been dead for 15 years. That night I sat up and cried and cried and cried and spoke to my mother, was I doing the right thing? Why had she left me? Anger spat out of me, and I cried more. I was so lonely with my secret, my feelings of guilt, why was I being punished like this.

My friend, Julie, was going to meet me at the hospital and we would go out that night, if I was OK. Because Ritchie was a drug user in prison, I was being put in a side ward and would be tested for HIV and then retested 3 months later.

The bus journey to the hospital took 55 minutes. I just wanted to get off. I didn't know what I wanted. I was led by anger.

I got to the hospital, got a side room, got some valium, was put to sleep and I felt empty...a void...loss. I woke up crying, my stomach was painful. Julie was there and I was allowed to go home at tea-time. I felt numb, like a robot. I got home, took more painkillers, bled and fell in and out of sleep. It was all over; I could put it behind me.

The next morning when I woke up, I just sat and stared at a wall and cried. My body was sore and my breasts still hurt. Julie was staying in Aberdeen and had to go home, but invited me up for Christmas. I said I would be in touch. I sat in the flat when she left for about 5 days eating, sleeping, crying, having panic attacks, and not getting dressed. I was in a pit of torture. I would not answer the phone or talk. I just felt angry and numb. The panic attacks were dreadful, but I deserved them, after what I had done. I eventually put all the baby clothes at the back of the wardrobe and the scan picture and decided I would move house after Christmas. I just couldn't bear to be in a house that Ritchie had tainted.

I went up to Aberdeen for Christmas and never got dressed for 4 days, just walked about in night clothes and ate food every waking moment. I hated myself. I loathed me. A part of me didn't want to go back to the flat, but I knew I had to. I managed to secure a private let in the centre of Edinburgh with a friend called Ann who took the occasional bit of smack. I was glad to be out of that old flat – once again another move, new walls, new life, past hidden.

I vowed to myself I would never go near another man. It was January 1989. I was not doing well. I was eating to fill the even bigger black void. I was stealing small items from shops and having major panic attacks. My doctor gave me valium and good old anti-depressants and referred me to a dietician.

I became a social recluse and just sat in the house and got bigger. My weight went up to about 20 stone. My back was starting to get sore and my legs, and my stomach was huge. I hated life. I hated people. I started to have suicidal thoughts.

I could not turn to my sister. She had enough of her own troubles, being a battered wife. I stayed clear of my dad and Tricia and my granny and granddad were not permanently in my life. I shared a flat with a drug addict and I was a food addict – great combination! I was desperate and very remorseful after the termination. I had no one to talk to. I just felt a deep hole of hollow and a great sadness and regret, and I wanted something to take it away.

I decided I had to go to Blackpool and find Ritchie (I still had to go back for a repeat blood test for HIV), and I just wanted him to make it alright. I was not thinking straight, but Julie and I took a train to Blackpool. We had a contact number from a phone bill I had that he had kept phoning. We called it and it was some probation social worker. We got an appointment to see her and she told us she was Ritchie's girlfriend's probation officer. She confirmed that Ritchie and the girl were back together and using drugs and it was wise for me to get a HIV test. She knew nothing about the pregnancy or me. She said she would contact Ritchie and ask if he wanted to meet with me. She was frightening me, all this talk about drug users (heroin) and prisons. She called me the next day and told me that Ritchie would not meet me, and to go home and get on with my life.

I felt so low, stupid, rejected and full of fear. I came back to Edinburgh and while waiting for the train I seriously considered throwing myself in front of it. What did I have and what did I have to look forward to, a life maybe with HIV. It was sheer torture. I had another 6 weeks to wait for the second test and it seemed like 6 years.

I just stayed in the flat and anaesthetized myself with food. I went for my second test in March in the City Hospital and spoke to someone about the implications if it was positive. I had an appointment to go back in 5 days to get the results personally. I am sure at this point I didn't care if I died, but I wanted it to be quickly, not slowly. Two people who I went to school with me and who had become drug users had died with AIDS and it took a period of time. I didn't want to suffer any more agony, I just wanted it over, should the result be positive. 80% of me had decided it would be positive and I went back for the results and it was negative.

CHAPTER 10

LIFE WITH ALCOHOLICS

It was May 1989, and I decided that I had to brush myself down and get on with it (the termination was being buried with food, panic attacks were still rife).

I started to visit my dad and Tricia again (I couldn't stop going back, it was like a magnet); so another mask was put on to face them to enable me to cope. They were drinking badly, Tricia was going on loads of binges with my dad and her kids were only 2 / 3 years old. I would meet them in the pub round from their house and sit and drink, not to excess, but sit and buy them drinks just to have company.

On one of these pub sessions, my dad introduced me to John Scott, who was 17 years older than me. (My dad told me to, "get in there, he is loaded with cash".) My first thought about John was nothing spectacular, but I felt drawn to him. I didn't find him attractive, but he spoke to me, and who would want me, the 'blob'. I suppose if my dad thought he was OK, then it would be OK to go out with him.

Once again, things moved very quickly. I moved in with him and his elderly mother. Within a month, John was off sick from his work (long-term). I was told it was stress but gradually realised it was alcoholism. I started to find empty vodka bottles hiding in drawers, cupboards, washing baskets. My life was dreadful with John. He was aggressive, paranoid and obsessed with jealousy. He would create situations and believe his paranoid thoughts. He would batter me and throw me out in the night. His mother, who I had become close to, tried to stick up for me, but he would shout and a couple of times hit her. For some strange reason, I told him about the termination and he would taunt me and shout murderer. A big part of me felt I deserved this life. I could handle it because I was familiar with it. (I couldn't really handle it; I was filling myself with food like an empty bucket.)

After being with John on and off for about 8 months, I managed to get myself a Housing Association flat. I had tried to get some sort of guidance from my dad, but his words were, "you made your bed, so lie in it". I got my little flat and managed to get a college course as a Nursery Nurse. The reasons I chose the Nursery Nurse course was I felt so tortured about the termination. My thinking was if I just go and work with kids I could make it better (it was sheer torture).

I did not cope well with the academic side of the work and some of the children on the placements I was put on commented about my weight. One person on the course in my class (who was, and had always been an acceptable size 10) said, "How did Sandra ever get a place on this course?

Just look at her." Also one of my tutors took me aside one day and said "What about your weight, Sandra?" It was very difficult for me, someone of 20 stone trying to run around after toddlers, sit on little chairs, bend and kneel. I was setting myself up for daily humiliation and torture and didn't realise it.

One summer job I got was with a little girl of 6 years old. She was so unhappy and came from a wealthy, dysfunctional family, two parents who were workaholics and had no time for her. The dad didn't want a daughter; well I knew how this felt. All I had to offer this little girl was empathy for her sadness. I didn't enjoy the job, as I was envious of her. She had material comfort and a room full of toys and a dependency on my dog and me. I knew I had nothing to offer her, I felt a fraud and false…But I did look after her with all those firework feelings inside me and was praised highly by her professional parents.

The course lasted until 1991. I skimmed through it. John stalked me, attacked me with a car key, stabbing my head, attempted to rape me, and my dad and Tricia still sat and drank with him.

My health was bad. I had constant thrush, back pain, knee problems, panic attacks and a bad bout of glandular fever. I was at the doctors like a second home. I could always be assured that I would come away from the doctors with my anti-depressants.

At college I made distant friends. I always kept people at a distance. I didn't want them to get to know the real me (whoever that was). John's mum died and I felt very sad. I started to go to the pub a lot more and started drinking more along with my dad and Tricia. I was staying 5 minutes walk from their house and I went on to meet John no. 2. He was 10 years older than me, divorced with 2 kids and a stonemason, and, surprise, surprise, a binge drinker. I lasted with John no. 2 for about 2 years. I moved house as Tricia and my dad kept appearing at my door looking for money for drink or leaving her two youngest kids with me for days on end, or my dad sleeping in my living-room due to her and my dad fighting. One time Tricia was in my house, her daughter had a kid with someone who broke into houses and stored his stolen stuff on the railway line. I stayed in a ground floor flat (due to my inability to manage stairs that well). This particular night I had about £200 cash in the house. Tricia was there and had seen this money. I hid it in my wardrobe. I also had a box of Roses chocolates someone had given me. Tricia pleaded with me to go out with her. So I did, I stayed out for 3 hours. When I got home, my flat had been broken into and my video, CDs, loads of things were gone. I phoned Tricia and my dad who sympathised.

The next day I went down to Tricia's daughter's house. There was a box of Roses chocolates sitting on top of the TV. When I got home the police told me that my video had been recovered on the railway line. Tricia set up the whole night – the chocolates, the video, it all slotted into place. They never found the money.

I knew I had to get out. I moved with John no. 2 into a flat that he got. He was never really physically abusive, just mental s**t, and unable to work because of the alcohol. I was still stealing, eating and drifting in and out of jobs. John's life was in the pub. My weight was 21 stone and I was a size 26. My health was bad and I was told by one of John's friends that I should be grateful, who would have me anyway.

Over the next few years, until I was 26, I had another 3 house moves, my weight was soaring up and I was desperate. My doctor referred me to an obesity clinic and I decided to go.

Self Help and Obsessions

Dr. Munro's clinic was for people who were morbidly obese. I was told that I was going to be put on a trial for a drug called Prozac (fluoxetine). I would not know if it was a placebo or the real thing, but it was being tested for an appetite suppressant. I gave it a shot. I thought I would feel some difference, but I felt nothing.

It was about this time that I read in a women's magazine about a woman who could not stop eating and a self-help group for compulsive overeaters. I could relate to what some of the article said and I took the number and called. My first ever meeting was in a cold church room and about 8 people were crammed into this little room. There were people of all shapes and sizes. One girl frightened me, she was a lot bigger than me, her breathing was heavy and she kept falling asleep. People spoke about different things, about feelings and thoughts, about the past, the present, what their eating habits were like and what they could or could not eat. I just sat there looking at the floor and listening, maintaining eye contact briefly if I was asked if I wanted to share anything. I realised I just listened. I got identification and a sense of belonging, but also a sense of fear that these people from all walks of life shared or used food like I did. I was going to go for 2 / 3 weeks and see how it went. We could exchange phone numbers but I declined at this point to give mine. I was still suspicious and did not want to commit to anything.

I still attended the obesity clinic and saw various doctors and patients who were on the same Prozac trial as me. Some of them were losing weight quickly and were coming out of their shells, grinning like the cat that had got the cream. The wonder drug was working for them, the solution. I was consumed with envy and the 'poor me' victim would go home and eat to comfort myself and punish myself as it was not working for me. Various different doctors that I had seen at the clinic told me the obesity was genetic and maybe I was just unlucky. I never felt a sense of believing or understanding at the clinic. I felt I was just dipping my toe in the water and so were the medics with the limited information they had about my condition. All I felt were more doors closing on me. But I wanted to be seen by my friends, social circle and family to be doing something about my weight. I wanted to be diagnosed with some big medical condition, under active thyroid or some new theory, so that I could get the go-ahead to continue eating. I was in so much denial about the compulsion that I didn't really understand or know the dependency I had on food, and I was not ready to give it up.

I was still going to the odd therapy session with the therapist. 5 years ago I sat for these sessions and would paint pictures and talk about happy childhood days with my mum and sister, never much about the current days or about what was going on in my life. My weight was never mentioned and I felt safe and secure with my therapist. I did pay a contribution fee to see her, but whatever time she gave me, was an escape or return to the happy, non-damaged little girl inside me.

I controlled the rules and the boundaries of these sessions and quickly picked up the jargon of the therapy world. If anything did get too uncomfortable, I would use the intellect of therapy jargon and I would go back to where I wanted. It was where I wanted to be and I could not let people in or see me at that stage of my life.

I wanted to have a baby with John no. 2, as I felt a baby would fill up the void in my life, and it would also ease the pain of the termination that still haunted me from the moment I opened my eyes to shutting them, but my food and drugs kept the pain controlled.

Having a baby with John was not going to be easy. He had a vasectomy 6 years previously and the NHS was not keen to reverse it. I went on and on and wouldn't stop. John eventually went to his doctor who asked him some medical questions about his health and was very negative about the NHS reversing his vasectomy.

We forgot to address the facts of his alcohol problem, my abuse of food and weight problem, the crazy co-dependant wreck of a relationship we were in. Never once did we sit down with each other and speak about being parents or what we had to offer a child. All I know is that I was like a child having a tantrum and wanted my way, but not for any of the right reasons. I wanted to make my past better to ease my pain of termination, to fill the void in my life and to prove to myself, my dad and Tricia that I could be a good mum and show them, through my child, all the things they should have done for me (rose-tinted glasses – magical thinking).

Over the next few months, John no. 2 and my life

just continued, him abusing alcohol, me abusing food, arguments, stealing, lying, trips to doctors for more anti-depressants, daily panic attacks, still going to the self-help group and listening, no eye contact, looking at the floor, no exchange of phone numbers. I was also still attending the obesity clinic and getting bigger.

At this stage, I was about 22 stone and I started to bath with an underskirt on, I couldn't face looking at my body. So each day I bathed it would take me an hour. I would fill the bath, get two bath towels, cover all mirrors with scarves or towels and get this white/grey waist underskirt. I had loads of anxiety about getting in and out of the bath. Most people went in baths to relax; I found the whole experience a terror and torture. I would pull the horrible waist slip over my breasts and it came down to my thighs. I would quickly wash and I would get one large towel and cover the top half of my body and then pull the underskirt down while still in the bath and dry myself quickly. I usually had thrush even coming out of my naval, and I would have sores at the tops of my legs and underneath my stomach where it hung over the pubic hair of my vagina, a big red sore rash would appear as it was getting no air or freedom from the folds of excess flesh that harboured these skin conditions. Creams, tablets, sprays were all prescribed to deal with the effects of the physical conditions that the obesity was causing. So it took me an hour just to get clean, but I accepted this.

I would not allow any full-length mirrors into my homes. If any were fixed to the walls, they would be covered with scarves, posters or pictures. A mirror from the neck up was all I wanted or could cope with.

When I went to bed with John no. 2 (which was not a lot), I would stay up and sleep or doze on the sofa. I would wear a black waist under-slip, a full nightdress that came down to my ankles and a floral light housecoat to bed. After we had sex, I would get up and put on clean pants and sleep in the living room. He used to joke with me that it would be easier getting into Fort Knox. We laughed, but the laughter hid my pain about my body issues. This was my life and I accepted it.

3 months after being referred to the vasectomy clinic, John no. 2 got the go-ahead to get a reversal at a private hospital in Glasgow and would get the operation paid for by the NHS. This was it, my life was going to change and in a year I would have a baby.

To fill the void that lay within me, I was not going out much. I didn't socialise, I was my own judge and jury before I went anywhere. I was unacceptable to me, so I didn't put myself in situations that meant meeting new people. I didn't have the skills to cope in social situations. I was both aggressive and unapproachable, or a people-pleaser (something my dad had moulded me into well). I didn't have any purpose or pattern in my life, just liked food. I would eat all day, never at set times and graze at food all day. Night times were the worst, I would make myself something to eat at 5 o'clock and be planning what I would eat at 7 o'clock. A lot of my thinking was taken up by food thoughts and this prevented me thinking or feeling other things. People could never understand how I was so big as I didn't eat much (their words), "And I had such a beautiful face if only I could lose weight". If one more f*****g person said that to me, I am sure I might have re-arranged their face. I still kept in contact with my friend, Julie, from the hostel and she was the only person who knew how some of me felt.

My granddad was now dead and I was a full time carer to my granny, which I resented. My aunts and uncles were leaving me to do their job and I could barely cope for myself. I surrounded myself with people who constantly needed me and performed my role well.

John no. 2 was not producing any sperm. The operation was not successful and it caused great arguments between us. I wanted out and decided to get myself a Cocker Spaniel dog, that I called Blue. I managed to get myself a job in a takeaway food shop (another compulsive overeater's paradise).

My dad and Tricia were still in my life and my 2 older step-brothers and step-sister were constantly at my house, just appearing at all times. They stole from me, they attacked me and the next day would expect me to continue as if nothing had happened, but this is what dysfunctional up-bringing does to one's self.

John no. 2 and I were at the end of the road. I managed to pass my driving test and held down my job for 3 months. I went away and bought a 2-bedroom house. I was 26 years old and 22 stone. The house was 5 miles away from my dad and Tricia and I wanted that. I also wanted to get away from John no. 2. So this was all done quietly.

I managed to buy a decent car and felt as if my life was going somewhere. It was 1994 and I finally felt ready to get away from my past (or so I thought). Before I did go, I had another argument with my step-brothers and when I got up the next day, they had scraped 'FAT' over my car bonnet with a knife. I felt angry and knew I had to get out. I felt so humiliated when I had to phone my insurance and taking it to the garage. Of course, it was never proven which one of them had done it. It cost £500+ for a re-spray.

I broke up with John, but didn't care. Thinking that new walls and different locations would heal the pain of the past, standing still but running away, I had done it in my mind for 22 years, so it was nothing new to me. Blue and I moved into my little semi-detached house, and life would be OK... (Magical thinking).

CHAPTER 11

ON MY OWN AND BITTERNESS

The first few months of moving into my home were taken up with the usual stuff that a new home demands, decoration, furniture, and garden stuff. It was August when I moved into my house and a big field was next to it for walking Blue.

I knew by moving to that house that it was too far for my dad and Tricia to come and annoy me, and only a handful of people knew where I stayed.

The obesity clinic was over and shutting down as there was not a demand for the service. I was still going to my self-help group with other compulsive overeaters and managed to form a couple of friendships and gave my phone number as a contact (I could always leave the answer-phone on when I didn't want to speak).

I had not been to therapy for a bout 9 months and my doctor was still giving me anti-depressants, which I would take for 3 months, stop and then restart.

My washing routine was still the same, and my 'going to bed cover up' routine was the same.

My body was now starting to ache if I lay in a certain position too long in bed. It would be my back or my hips, my knees were also getting very sore and my skin was still chaffing from excess flesh and not getting aired.

I lasted in total 6 months in the takeaway. I couldn't stand for any long periods and was so hung-over with food in the morning and trying to get myself ready with my daily washing ritual, I physically or mentally could not manage to work. Up until April 1995, I had a life of caring for my granny, my dog, eating, sleeping, and patting myself on the back for getting away from dad & Tricia. I was physically removed but the demons were raw each night. I would come home, close the curtains, lay food on my coffee table and eat until I was anaesthetized, and fall into a sleep on the sofa and wake about 12.30am. I would then stagger up to bed taking a chocolate bar for comfort and wake up in the morning, come down to the living-room and pick up all the wrappers and empty packets lying on the floor in a fog of denial.

I was still in touch with my sister briefly. She had got out of her marriage and went on to have a kid with someone else. We didn't meet much but kept in touch via the telephone. She would tell me snippets of my dad and Tricia's life and I never commented.

I went back to college part-time for basic course core skills. I was on incapacity benefit, as I was not fit for work, physically or mentally. I had a lot of literature from the self-help group that I would pick up now and then and skim over it. I can always remember getting up one day, it was April 1995 and my weight was 23½ stone. I was 27 years old and I felt dreadful. I decided that I had to do something, I could not continue like this. The pain I was feeling felt as raw as losing my mum or losing my baby. I knew my life could not go on like this. I decided I would go to a meeting 3 times a week. I would go back to therapy, I would eat 1,000 calories a day and walk most days and weigh myself when I felt like it.

I went through sugar withdrawal. I cried for about 2 whole days, I didn't go out for 4 days. I was nervous and shaky. My comfort, friend and cage were away. I felt naked and exposed.

I went back to therapy and started to see a different therapist. We started to talk about deeper things, food, and body image…the black hole, different things. Sometimes I had to go twice a week.
I was not on anti-depressants and I was going to meetings 3 times a week.

I was sticking to the 1,000 calories a day and my mind was not clouded or possessed with food. I still didn't have the understanding or feeling of being hungry or full, but I stuck to my eating plan and my clothes started to get loose. People started to tell me how well I looked (I felt very uncomfortable, I had 22 years of being told how bad I was, I couldn't cope with the good words). I was practising eye contact and a path towards commitment, respect and honesty towards people, on a daily basis. I didn't look at my plan as needing to lose 10 or 12 stone; I just did it on a daily basis.

I tried to create balance in my life and keep my life simple (this was not easy). I was used to dramas; highs / lows, giving all this up was not easy, avoiding people, places, things that made me uncomfortable was not easy either. I was looking inside myself with support from other group members, therapy and tools I picked up. I wrote a daily diary of my feelings (not my food). I took a past inventory of myself, I practiced honesty and attempted to make amends for the wrong I had done in my life. I was trying to find me again, the person I had buried under food, and it was not easy…But at this point in my life I didn't want to give into the big black hole. I was in daily recovery and grateful.

CHAPTER 12

MARRIAGE AND ME

By the time of November 1995, I had committed 7 months to this daily plan of my new life. I was 17½ stone and a size 18. I still felt emptiness in me and I had done lots of intense internal therapy. It left me with me. What did I want from life? This was not some miraculous transformation I was having, this was a painful look inside me and looking in at what I had become, lost and buried. Some days the feelings and fears felt so powerful that I wanted to run back to the food or the people or places that hid me from me. I was trying to make my life simple and it was not easy for someone who had been a compulsive caretaker of other people, a thief, a liar, and a people pleaser. I felt like I was left with an empty shell (which I was, me). But I kept reading the literature of the self-help group and listening to others share their experiences. It took me 5 years of sitting and listening but I kept going back and it was paying off. The only thing I found very uncomfortable and difficult was when people praised me. It wasn't a feeling or understanding I was comfortable with, so I quickly diverted away from it.

I didn't really know what direction or where my life was going but I wanted some happiness and started to reply to date ads in lonely-hearts columns. I was still not confident enough to go out socialising. One person replied to my ad who caught my interest was Bill, who was 11 years older than me and stayed in a fishing village 30 miles from me. Bill was divorced and had 4 kids. We spoke on the phone a lot and the phone can hide a lot and fabricate a lot.

After speaking on about 4 occasions, we decided to meet. I had a lot of anxiety about this. I also felt that bit more acceptable as I was just over 17 stone and not being judged either by society or myself (the washing ritual was still there). I met Bill for a meal and we got on well. He was about 6' and a few stone overweight. We decided to keep in touch and meet again. I did find it quite strange that Bill would phone me at strange times and sometimes through the night, but I comforted these thoughts by saying this is what people must do if they like each other. I did have a strange feeling in my stomach of fear and excitement when I was speaking to Bill but I felt connected to him.

At this point I got a job in a ladies' clothes shop (for outsize clothing). I fitted the bill and it was quite creative work. I mostly worked on my own, which was OK. I met up with Bill a few more times, nothing physical happened but I liked him.

It was when I went to his flat for the third time; I found empty whisky bottles under the bed. I felt sad and at first denied it was happening again. Is that all I would ever get in life, an alcoholic? Is that all I deserved? I had the qualifactions, training and masks to deal with them but deep down they frightened me. I confronted Bill down the telephone, not very constructively, and he told me he had lost his family, job and himself and had been in treatment and relapsed. This was another person that needed me. I could comfort him, but I was reserved.

It was the start of December 1995 and I was going on a night out for Christmas with a friend. It was the 2nd of December. I had known Bill for 6 weeks and it felt like a lifetime. Nothing intimate happened between us (I don't think Bill was capable), but I kept being a compulsive caretaker to him, coming away with feelings of sadness, frustration, and emptiness. My eating was creeping back up, my meetings were slipping, and I was slipping back into denial.

On the night out, this is where I met my son's father. I was in a nightclub and felt OK. I had made a special effort with my hair and make up. I did not go out socialising much and the club was very busy. I bumped into James, my future husband; my first thoughts of James were negative (it was that of all men). He spoke to me and I was trying to make the effort to respond. I was not drinking as I was driving. James was 29 years old. A driver and divorced, he stayed with his mum and brother and he had a son of 9 to his previous wife. I invited him back to my house for coffee. My house was homely and I must have fitted his agenda as when he sat on one of my sofas, he looked like he fitted in. We spoke and decided to meet the next day. We went bowling and I liked him, but I was also frightened. James spoke of his family; I hid mine ashamed and frightened. If they were brought into the conversation, then I might be judged as part of them and I had worked so hard to be free of them. Things happened very quickly for James and me. We both had neediness but mine was a lot higher than his. Bill was still in the background and I couldn't break away from him. He was like a magnet always drawing me back with his helplessness and my compulsive care taking.

James knew nothing of Bill until he moved in with me, 3 weeks after we met, and as Bill was phoning me at all hours. I told James briefly about Bill (I was just reliving father – daughter dysfunction with Bill but couldn't see it). Julie, my friend, thought James was OK and this was important to me. My sister who I met briefly thought he was OK and I felt happiness. My granny called him a country bumpkin as he lived out of town, but she seemed to warm to him.

James took me to meet his mum and she had a family home, all the things I had ever wanted. She was pleasant and welcoming. She was of a similar build to me, overweight but holding it OK. James' mum and dad were divorced. James was quite a reserved person and quiet and sensitive. I was the opposite, controlling, aggressive, outspoken and fronted a mask of being capable. James showed me affection, which I always felt uncomfortable with. He would buy me flowers or want to hold my hand in public places. I could not handle this. It's funny how you are concerned with something and still manage to escape it by looking at the floor or pretending you need the loo or need to make an urgent call, all these methods supported me in not having to respond to James' affection. After I had been with James for 5 weeks, I told him I was a compulsive eater. (This compulsive overeating terminology was still new to me and I was still coming to terms with that disease I had.) James nodded his head like a lost puppy as if I was speaking some foreign language (in a way I was). He told me it was OK and he understood (wrong thing to say). If it was OK, then I could go back to my world of food because I sure needed it, all this acceptance, change, and displays of affection were freaking me out and the only friend I could turn to was food. James' work was not steady; one week he would work 50 hours and the next 6 hours. I was still working in the clothes shop, still there and I was up 2 dress sizes, but I was in a bubble of organising a wedding. Bill's calls were fading, but once a fortnight I would still visit him (without James knowing).

Our wedding was to be 11th May 1996. On Valentine's Day, 2 weeks after James had asked me to marry him, we went away for the weekend. I did not feel well; I was so tired and coming down with a cold, but still wrapped up with wedding books and food.

My whole life had changed dramatically. Since December 2nd 1995 (even at this stage no mention of love from me) James expressed his feelings to me. My way of giving him affection back was to cook, clean, care for him (mother him). That's all I had to give because something else loved me and I loved it, food.

When we got home from that weekend, I did a pregnancy test (4 actually) and they were positive. I was so happy but frightened. My whole life was going in a different direction, but I was content to go along with it. As I had food, I was in the pits of my compulsion again and what had started out as a size 22 wedding dress became a size 28. James liked food and was a couple of stone overweight. We ate a lot of takeaways and his eating habits were erratic as he worked through the night sometimes. We were funding the wedding ourselves (mostly me), but I had to keep up the show, for my family and James' family. I did not want any cracks. The wedding was costing about £6,000 and I could ill afford it. I got into debt, loans, overdrafts, etc.

At this stage as I was pregnant and was eating for 2, I could eat what I wanted. I was getting bigger and bigger. I invited all my dad's side of the family to my wedding and my dad and Tricia. (I had a great fear about my dad and Tricia showing me up, getting drunk, arguing or Tricia, when eating, taking her false teeth out). This frightened me. I sent them all invitations. My dad and Tricia never replied. James had not even met my dad, but my sister told me my dad was coming to give me away (he would

be proud of me). I had 2 bridesmaids and 2 flower girls. James had his best friend, Alec, as best man.

On the day of the wedding everything was the usual stress, flowers arriving, hairdresser, and cars. The plan was my dad was to come to the house, go in the bride car with me and Tricia would meet him at the church. A part of me did not want my dad and Tricia there as I had a fear of them sabotaging my day.

My sister called my Auntie, my dad's sister and came off the phone hysterical. My dad was not coming because Tricia wasn't getting in a wedding car. Well 'stiff upper lip' for me; time to comfort my sister. No time for my sadness or let down or anger. Deal with the practicalities of someone giving me away. My next-door neighbour's husband would do it. My sister was still having her drama over it. I brushed it under the carpet and dealt with it. A part of me was relieved that they would not be there, as I was fearful of the shame they would bring me. James and I got married in my size 28 dress and three months pregnant.

The day went like it should have, apart from my

dad's family offering me words of sympathy for him letting me down. I took it in my stride. At one point at my wedding reception, I remember sitting alone, feeling like an outsider looking in. I quickly shrugged this feeling off, but it was pretty powerful. I did not care about my weight that day, as I was allowed to be overweight in my mind as I was pregnant and still in denial about my eating. James and I had decided (mostly me) that we would make a fresh start; we were going to rent my house out to pay the mortgage and cover some debts the wedding had built up. James bought a flat with my input and control in the same village as Bill and we moved in after the wedding (I still felt the need to have people with alcohol problems in my life as I was not giving up my care-taking role and it took me away from standing still but running away).

We moved into the flat in Fife. I was 4 months pregnant and moved on from wedding magazines to mother and baby magazines and, of course, biscuits and sweets at my side.

CHAPTER 13

BIRTH AND DISABILITY

My granny did not come to the wedding. She was not well enough. She was happy I was married and going to have a baby. I was about six months pregnant and I had my second scan. I didn't feel maternal, I felt practical, going to buy baby clothes, equipment. I felt comfortable with my body, not physically comfortable, but in my mind acceptable to be big. I was about 23 stone and 6 months pregnant. At my second scan the doctors requested that I had another scan in a few weeks, as they could not see the baby's spine. (I knew I was being punished for the termination.) Those 2 weeks were dreadful, a haze of food and isolation for me. I slept on my own. The demons were coming back to haunt me. I locked James out. We had only been in our nice new flat for 4 months and it was all going wrong yet again (victim mask). It turned out the baby was fine; it was the way it was laying.

I was frightened, I didn't want to be in Fife anymore, so six weeks before the baby was due, we moved back to my house in Edinburgh. Once again running and changing the walls and location because I was frightened, frightened of me, of motherhood, of a baby...But like the wedding feeling, I quickly dismissed this and ate to comfort me.

I was also not comfortable with the closeness of marriage and the commitment it demanded from me. A compulsive overeater and marriage, no competition – the food always won.

Edward, my son, was due to be born on my late mother's birthday (25th October), but because he was getting fed huge amounts of ice-cream, chocolate, takeaways, I don't think he wanted to come out to the cold world. A few days past my due date, I was seen at the hospital by a female Mexican doctor who told me that I was very overweight and could have blood clots and die. (Once again humiliated and punished for being grossly overweight). By now I was past caring if I died, but she did put the fear of hell into me. It was decided I would go in on 7th November, two weeks after my due date and they would induce me. I went home and stayed home for the next ten days eating, sleeping and being uncomfortable. On the 7th of November still nothing started, so with my neat bag packed and my mother and baby magazines (one article I read was about post-natal depression, I read it with care and kept thinking of it obsessively but I tried to put it to the back of my mind), I went to the hospital. When I got to hospital, my waters were manually broken and I was given a gel to start me.

Eight hours later I thought I was in full-blown labour. I was only 3cms dilated the next day. I was given more gel and was having painful contractions. The young midwife got the doctor and it turned out that Edward was in distress. I was quickly whisked away to theatre to have an emergency c-section. The doctors seemed angry that they could not freeze me with a spinal epidural due to my weight, but they were also scared to knock me out using an anaesthetic. Because of my weight, it was extremely risky and, to top it all, the Mexican's doctor's words went through my head, "You could die". Very quickly, my husband was ushered out and I was knocked out.

Edward James was born at 3.30pm on 8th November 1996 and I woke up at 8.30pm with a breathing mask on me and oxygen at my side. I felt dreadful. Edward was brought to me but I could not hold him as I was in too much pain, physically and mentally. I did not feel anything, even as I drifted in and out of sleep. I thought of the food trolley outside my ward in the corridor.

The next few days in hospital were dreadful. I felt very low and I wanted out of this motherhood thing. I could hardly care for me, let alone a baby. But once again, I pulled out one of my coping masks for James, my husband, for his family and all my friends that came to visit me.

Three days after Edward was born, I felt nothing. I felt numb, empty, and void. I had nothing to give. I burst out crying for three whole hours. A nurse, no more than 20 years old, told me it was the baby blues. I knew whatever this was; it was more than baby blues. I signed myself out of hospital that day. I felt nothing for my baby. I went home and each day district nurses came to inject me for blood clots in my legs. My midwife came to see me and I still tried to keep up the show. Edward was a good baby, no crying, just fed, slept, and made little noises. My sleep was dreadful. My thoughts were worrying. I wanted to run away. I wanted to hide Edward. I felt shame, guilt and if Edward cried, I got very stressed out.

After being home for six / seven days, I could not cope anymore. About 1.00am on a Friday morning I called an emergency GP who spoke to me and sent an ambulance. I felt such guilt, relief and sadness at leaving my baby and husband behind. James knew nothing until I woke him and told him I was going to a psychiatric hospital. He cried. I couldn't help him. Edward slept.

Once again I was a failure, coping out. I went to the hospital. I just lay in a bed, empty and wanting to be dead (really dead). I lay in the hospital ward for 5 days and James came and visited me and cried. All our dreams and parenthood were taken away from us. Edward went to James' mum. I did not want to see him. I could not cope. It was decided that I was suffering from post-natal depression and eventually the nursing staff realised that I had an infected wound, a form of the MRSA bug, which needed swift medical attention.

The Professor from the maternity hospital came up to visit me personally and apologised for the birth complications. I found out that Edward was also resuscitated for 8 minutes. He apologised for the Mexican doctor.

I had to be moved to a mother and baby unit in the hospital and my wound was dressed and cleaned three times a day. The smell of an infected wound and being 14 stone overweight did not help. I was a wreck, but I was secure in my mind, Edward was safe in my mother-in-law's hands. James was visiting me every day for 4 – 5 hours. I felt smothered and felt I did not have the time to be ill as I was constantly reassuring him that everything would be OK. How the f**k would everything be OK? I asked myself when I was in a psychiatric hospital. Physically and mentally out of it and my baby was with another woman.

After I had Edward, I had a lot of incontinence, urine and bowel. My legs were in constant pain and I could barely stand or walk any distance. I was on two different kinds of anti-depressants and eventually anti-psychotic drugs as my depression was slipping into a purple psychosis. Twice I was sectioned under the Mental Health Act. I was on various painkillers and tranquillisers. Every night when I shut my eyes, my last thoughts were of my baby, how I felt I had abandoned him. He would come and visit me twice a week. All I felt was guilt and relief when he went away. I felt edgy and uncomfortable around him. James was not working at this time and bills and debts were mounting up.

Eight weeks after I had Edward, it was decided that he would come into hospital with me. I was frightened. The plan was a nurse would shadow me everywhere, and I mean everywhere. Edward had a place in the nursery and slept there. I slept in my single room (with hoards of food, my weight was 25½ stone). I resented the nurse shadowing me, but I needed her to make me feel safe. Every time Edward cried, that ugly f*****g demon came into my head from childhood "shut him up" (just like I was). What if I batter him or harm him? The intelligent woman inside me told me I would never do this. Every time he smiled at me, I cried with sadness and inability to bond. I was trying to care for him practically, change, feed, sleep, bath, that's about the best I could give and please believe me, that was a struggle.

My body was failing me; I could not bend or kneel. An occupational therapist came to see me and gave me a stick to help pick things up. I also got a walking stick to help me around. I felt humiliated, but not enough to give up food.

One day, in February 1997, I had a bad day and spoke to a male nurse on the ward and said that I could not cope with this way of life and was considering putting Edward up for adoption. He said powerful, impactful words back to me, "Only a good mother would consider something like that" and stated that I must have cared about Edward. I wanted to care, but just did not know how. Those words helped and comforted me more than any of the anti-depressants.

Each week there would be a ward round to discuss your care plan. This involved the Consultant Psychiatrist, nursing staff, medical students, social workers, health visitors, and occupational therapists. In one of these meetings was the patient, who always got an allocated time to be present. They asked me about my eating habits. I looked at the ground with shame; words failed me. I felt like some monkey in a cage, some experiment. I wanted them to tell me the answers to my eating. I wanted to say I was the reverse to the anorexics / bulimics on the ward, but didn't have the insight or vocabulary – This was 1997; "compulsive eating" was left behind, still in its prime. It was suggested that I be added onto a list to see the outpatients' clinic that dealt with eating disorders (mostly bulimia / anorexia), and while I was there, I could see a dietician. (Funny how all these words, dietician / disease can all spell "die", as that's how I felt when they took away my crutch.)

My granny was still alive at this time, and was very worried about me, but powerless to do anything. She probably missed my company and the care I gave her when I was well, but I couldn't give anything. I visited her on a day pass and tried to hide a lot of what was going on. I didn't want to feel a failure or burden her.

Life on the ward was very different from the outside world, and I formed many friendships. One girl I made friends with, Jenny, had suffered from anorexia for eight years. She was about 19 and was in and out of hospital for the best part of eight years, usually with a drip attached to her arm. Some of the nursing staff were very unkind in their words about her, stating that she wasted resources and NHS time and money. She went out one day on a day pass, booked into a hotel and killed herself – no more waste of resources!

People with different eating disorders in the hospital tended not to talk about them or their feelings. Maybe it was the powerful denial that eating disorders hold, or maybe fear. I know for me, first and foremost, it is denial.

My time on the ward was coming to an end. It was March 1997 and I was going home with Edward and James three times a week, staying over 1 / 2 nights, always safe in the knowledge that I could go back to the hospital if it was too much. My discharge was coming near. I had an occupational therapist go to my house and assess my needs. I needed help with getting in and out of the bath, a monkey pole to help me out of bed, and an urgent request to the local housing that I be re-housed in a one-level, ground floor house or flat. I also had a social worker that got Edward a place in day care (childminder), 3 days a week. I also wanted a visit from a disability assessment doctor to assess my mobility. When he came, he asked me a series of questions and asked me to demonstrate some skills of working. He told me that I had mobility restriction and osteoporosis arthritis in my knees due to the wear and tear of being morbidly obese. I was now registered disabled at the ripe old age of 30 years.

A mother to a 5-month-old baby and a wife to my husband, a very limited walker to my dog, Blue and did I stop eating. NO! I didn't really have that much to stop for (why me, poor me, anger, let down, no self-esteem, more punishment) …More food…My friend, my comfort, my drug.

CHAPTER 14

MOTHERHOOD & COPING

Some of the things I had been taught on the nursery nurse course came in useful to me when caring for Edward, but everything took twice as long. Here I was at home with a young baby, gaga out of my head with anti-depressants, and my body f****d (morbidly obese). The mother and baby magazines failed me. Support was in place for me. Edward went to day-care three full days a week, and if I couldn't cope, my mother-in-law took him. She was very organised and practical and couldn't understand how I could not pull myself together as she had five kids (her kind, compassionate words to me). It was like a battle between her and me over Edward. If I dressed Edward in a suit she didn't like, she would change him into something she liked. If I didn't want him to eat certain foods (e.g., meat), she would just give him it when I left, always undermining me. She wasn't a nasty woman, she was someone who had a lot of anxiety, energy and came across as very capable and in control. She would run around after everyone, cook, clean, she actually had an obsessively clean house. Whenever James and I argued, he would walk away and then start cleaning the house, so as we argued a lot, we had quite a clean house!

James had another son about 11 years old to his

first wife and the CSA were chasing him for money. He was in and out of driving jobs and work was not steady. Our debts were mounting up. James decided to run his own cleaning company for a while. I helped out with some office stuff, calls, paperwork, but my health was failing me. I was not sleeping well. Edward was a good sleeper. I was sleeping separately from James. I was caring for Edward the best that I could practically, but still did not feel the bond. He was nearly one. I was still trying to care for my granny who had become ill. I resented my uncles and aunts. They would visit my granny every three / four months and leave all the care to a good neighbour called Mabel and me. My granny told me in 1997 that she had bleeding from the back passage and she was scared to die. I comforted her and told her mum would be waiting for her. She knew she was dying. When I eventually got her to go to hospital, she was diagnosed with bowel cancer, the same illness that had robbed her of her daughter in 1973. I had the civility to inform my aunts and uncles who put on a great show for the hospital and the hospice staff.

My granny was happy I was married and had a baby. If ever Edward cried when I visited her, she said, "Just dip his dummy in jam or lemon curd that will shut him up." (Maybe that's what method was used to shut me up into a compulsion for 35 years).

I had many aggressive confrontations with my

aunts and uncles – the devoted, loyal family that were never there for me or my granny. Even on my granny's deathbed, they got her to change her will. I didn't care about wills or death money. I am sure I was in a bit of denial about my granny's illness. One day in October, I was sitting reading the local paper. I hadn't been to see my granny for about four days, and I did something I had never done before, I went to the death column, my granny's death. Not one of those b*****ds could have the human respect to tell me. The control freaks that had kept my sister and me in silence about my mum's death, had now kept me in silence about my granny's. I was not a little girl anymore. I was 31 nearly. I cried a little for my granny, but was consumed with anger. I went to my granny's funeral with my sister, James and Julie, my friend. We all walked into the church with our heads held high. They all looked at the floor, not one of them could maintain eye contact with me (long may they continue to hold their heads down in shame). After the church, one uncle (who had taken me in when I was 13) came over and spoke to me. My sister and I went to the grave and forced our way forward with a red rose to lie on my granny's coffin. My dad (who I had not seen for 2 years) turned up at the grave half p****d. Seemingly, he went back to the hotel with them and bad mouthed me, all for the sake of free drink. After my granny's death, my marriage was falling apart. We were constantly arguing. I was eating worse than ever. I had very bad bowel and bladder incontinence. My sister was back on the scene for a while and I started, once again, to play my role of Mrs. Strength and mother her (she took my granny's place). My sister ended up having a nervous breakdown and getting hospitalised in the same hospital where I had two episodes of distress. My sister's kids were between their father and me. I was constantly going up to the hospital and trying to care for Edward who was about 18 months old. My sister was completely out of it.

Round about this time, I got an appointment for the eating disorders clinic. I had seen a male psychiatrist there on my first consultation. We went over old ground, family history, etc. He told me after speaking for about 30 minutes that I could have six sessions and to write all my food down that I ate. (Well here was Mr. Magic, a compulsion I had for 28 years, he was giving me six sessions and wanted me to write down everything I ate, did he want me to feel the humiliation and shame any further than I already did by putting it in a f*****g notebook...Six sessions, after all the years of body-hate-body-abuse... All it warranted was six sessions ...F**k him, another barrier up... No more appointments for me). More food. (I didn't realise these people were in the dark, and didn't seem to want to seek the light). I wanted solutions. I decided I was not going back, but started going back to my self-help group. I was not judged. I was not asked where or why I had left. I was at my biggest, but I was not ridiculed or humiliated. I was accepted by others (not myself at this stage). I also decided I would go back to therapy. Things were not good in any areas of my life and I had to get my act together.

Edward was nearly 2. I was starting to get some confidence and felt comfortable with him and enjoyed some days with him. He was in day-care nursery now. (My dad and Tricia had never seen him. I would never expose him to any dealings with them.) I felt strongly protective of him. James and I never had much physical contact with each other. We were just like two flatmates (or hates) that shared a flat. We had been re-housed to a disabled flat, all on one level. I was just under 26 stone. It was 1998. The summer months were dreadful. My care consisted of daily showers (mirrors covered), skin creams for thrush, rash (body covered quickly with clothes), and sweat would be dripping off me when I came out of the shower. I had two sets of clothes I usually wore, blue trousers (elasticated waist) or a purple skirt (still have that skirt), size 32. My medication consisted of 2 anti-depressants, painkillers, and the odd sleeping pill or tranquiliser. To get myself ready took about 1½ hour, and then I had to deal with Edward. Sometimes, if my health was really bad, I would get homecare visits from social services. (I would always do my hair nice everyday and my make-up. After all, thousands of people told me I had a beautiful face, if only I could lose the weight. If only!)

CHAPTER 15
DIVORCE AND ROCK BOTTOM

It was 1999 and James and I were going our separate ways. We were arguing all the time. A compulsion to food and a marriage were just not working. We never did anything together. We just ate, slept, cared for Edward and slept in separate rooms. James would go away for days on end, either to his mum's or friends. (I used to pretend in my head I would stay with him until Edward was 16, no divorce for me, no failure like my mum and dad.) My weight was hitting 26 stone and I could hardly wipe myself after a bowel movement because of the bulk of flesh, so after a bowel movement I would always shower (still not enough humiliation or shame to confront this compulsion). I started to go back to therapy and had a good therapist who I spoke to about the demons of my past that tortured me now. (I paid privately for therapy.) I also went to the self-help group weekly. I used to get comfort from people who were bigger than me (and there were some), and I also envied people who were thinner or had recovered. (I wanted what they had, but without doing the footwork.)

James and I separated in 1998, but came back and forward.

I had another 4-week stint at the psychiatric hospital in early February 1999. I knew I had to catch a grip but how did I get there.

On the day of 31st August 1999, when Lady Diana died, James had been back for a few months (there was no physical contact for about a year between us), we just could not make that final ending. But on this day, we had a really violent argument (James never once hit me). He said to me, "Look at the state of you. Who would screw you?" I stood up (I still had a little pride and dignity) and retaliated with, "Not you anyway!" The shouting and screaming went back and forth, and I got the police to remove him. That was the last day James and I spent with each other. I lodged divorce proceedings. I knew whatever we had was never going to return, and Edward was not going to be exposed to living with two screaming angry adults.

In this year James' best friend and best man at our wedding had died aged 36, of CJD. We both found this hard but James walked about and got on with life like a block of ice. Whenever I tried to talk about it to him, he would divert the conversation to something else.

I was s**t scared of being left with Edward, who was now 2½, but I did have support. I had day-care, Julie was around and my sister was a phone call away (even though she had her own problems). James took Edward once a week and stayed with his mum (Edward's granny never stopped seeing him). I, at this stage, was still using the walking stick and aid to help me. I could not lie too long in bed, as it was very uncomfortable with my weight. I remember thinking how lonely I was. I sat in night after night with my cupboards and fridge loaded up with my friend and enemy, my comfort and crutch, and when Edward went to bed, sat and ate. James' words rang in my ears, "Look at you. Who would screw you?" James was giving me no money for Edward, so I was on benefits.

In September 1999, a friend came to stay with me as they were in-between houses and it was company for me. In October 1999, I put an ad in a dating magazine and got a reply from, believe it or not, another James. I did not have any confidence to go out and meet someone face-to-face, but I did feel ready to meet someone, as I had really been separated from Edward's dad for 18 months, even though we shared a flat back and forth...But nothing ever went on between us. I knew the final departure on 31st August was final.

I was surprised how well I was coping with Edward and how I had grown to love him. He was my world (and it had taken me a long time to get those feelings.) I could tell with my protectiveness towards him. The stories I read him, the kisses we gave each other and the little child he allowed me to be, he allowed me to open a door that was so cruelly taken away. (I had not seen my dad or Tricia for six years, apart from my granny's funeral, where I had seen my dad briefly.) Fate blew another funny blow in this year. Tricia had got in touch with my sister. My dad had been rushed into hospital with a brain haemorrhage. I was to go and visit him (the dutiful daughter). I felt fear, fear of going back, fear of the confrontation, and fear of the awkwardness. I felt obligated to go and angry. I visited my dad twice on the first visit. Tricia's sisters were there with their daggers at Maureen and me; this is hostility I could do without. But this was a time to fill up their day, sitting in a waiting area, pretending to be concerned about my dad and gossiping about all the other people and probably about Maureen and me when our backs were turned. Tricia was once again controlling the drama and show. Nobody was allowed to see my dad without her being present. When my sister and I went in the doctors were doing their rounds and one of them started to talk to me about my dad's condition. She gave me a dirty look and pushed herself forward and said she was Mrs. Gallagher. (I think the doctor thought I was his wife. Overweight / obesity does seem to make you look older.)

I did not feel a lot for my dad, truth be told. I just wanted to get out of there. I didn't feel much, just numb and angry. I was angry with my dad for allowing drink, fags and lifestyle to put him there. (A part of me was frightened maybe my addiction might put me there.) Tricia mentioned at this point to my dad that he would need to stop drinking (supportive words). My dad was semi-awake. I believe he had keyhole surgery. He nodded his head like a puppy and agreed with her. I didn't stay long. The conversation was strained and the negativity and hostility. I just made my excuses and I left. It was a stranger in the bed, not my dad.

I got on with my life and did not let the hospital visit affect me. I knew that there was no going back for me. I started speaking to James on the phone (James no. 2). We got on great on the phone and spoke about music, the past, and the future. We had 3 / 4 hour conversations over a period of a month. Edward's dad's visits were getting less and less. He would say he would pick Edward up and just not turn up. (I half expected this.) I felt hurt and sad for Edward, especially when he promised to come to his 3rd birthday and didn't even bother to come or phone to wish him Happy Birthday.

I was very nervous about meeting James No. 2 and suggested we put it off for a bit and just speak on the phone. (I was frightened he would judge me by my weight and reject me.) We spoke for about five weeks before meeting and met at the beach, one winter night in November 1999. The build-up to it was frightening. Edward was going to a friend's house and I was taking Blue with me to meet him. (I maybe thought Blue would lick me to death with affection if it all went pear shaped.) I made a special effort with my hair and make-up and went to the overpriced shop (only shop) that would accommodate my size and bought a £80 outfit. (I always felt anger at this shop for ripping big people off; making money out of people's misery was big business.) I, in my past days, stole a few things out of these shops for a few different reasons, one, anger at being exploited, and two; I wasn't worthy of buying nice clothes or making myself attractive (self-esteem zero). I managed to go and meet James. He was tall and slim about 6' and going bald. He was very polite (thought he was just being kind because of my weight, my thinking). We sat on a bench with Blue sniffing the sand and got on well, but we were bloody freezing. We decided to go back to mine for a coffee (James stayed 25 miles away). It was strange sitting speaking to a guy in my home, meeting him for the first time without alcohol or loud music or my dad & Tricia's dysfunctional friends. James left about 12.30am. He gave me a kiss on the cheek and said he would phone me tomorrow. I liked him, I got on well with him, but I still had that thought at the back of my head that this would go wrong and a reservation mask in case I got rejected. I topped myself up with some food and went to bed and fell asleep.

I woke the next day having had 30 years of compulsive behaviour and thoughts. I expected James to call me first thing in the morning. By the time I picked Edward up at 1.00pm, he was written off, f*****g b*****d, just used me (what for a cup of tea, pretty long trip to come for a cup of tea), didn't really like him anyway. His entire negative thought pattern was going through my head. Because I had never shown much civility or affection from me for who I really was and in these intense 3 / 4 hour conversations with James no. 2, I had given away some of me. It was easy to write him off as this helped with the rejection I felt. I had a food binge, calm and sedated. It was now about 3.00pm. I looked at the stupid outsize clothes I had bought yesterday and threw them in the wardrobe (like a 4 year old having a tantrum). At 4.00pm James phoned. All the negative thoughts went. I explained to him I thought he wouldn't phone. James and I became a couple in December 1999.

My sister, at this time, was keeping in touch with my dad. She would also refer to the sexual abuse she experienced. She would never speak about it, but refer to it and felt very sad when she referred to it and would dismiss it quickly. I told her there was no f*****g way I would ever confront them. I wasn't going to let myself be exposed and let him sell himself through his neglect and abuse of us for drink. I said I would go down the proper channels and that was the Police, but the ball was in my sister's court. I couldn't do the foot or mouth work for her. (I had been the spokeswoman / child all my life, but this one was not my call.)

It was December 1999 and life with me, James and Edward was OK. James and I saw each other 3 – 4 times a week. Edward's dad and I were near to the final stages of divorce. He was not seeing Edward. He met me in December 1999 to talk about the home, debts, but not

Edward. I met him on my own. I could tell he had met someone else (another Sandra and me a James - freaky!). I paid him money, which my granny had left me and I got left the flat and the debts. I was not fit to work; my body would not allow it. My day was taken up with caring for Edward and my complex health needs due to my weight and compulsion. We were ready to go into 2000 and that Christmas was nice (apart from us all having the flu). James bought me a beautiful diamond ring and Edward a small guitar. He was going to teach Edward the guitar. He played it himself and he was very calming with Edward.

We spoke about how we would be with Edward as I had the insight not to expose him to too much change. James was like a playmate to him. We never hid our relationship from him, but would let him know when we felt he was ready. James was very complimentary to me, and I found this very uncomfortable. He would compliment me on my make-up and hair, and my weight didn't seem to affect him (but it did me). He liked big women (but did I?).

Edward's granny still kept in contact with him and overnight visits. (I felt very bad about my divorce and also that I had a boyfriend. I felt like I was being my mother all over again; divorce – boyfriend – eating disorder). But Edward was my life.

Towards the end of 1999, I was still going to

therapy and a friend of mine had had an operation, as she had been morbidly obese. She had gone from 27½ stone to 13½ stone. I was going to go to my GP and find out if I could get it done. I didn't want my life to continue like it was (morbidly obese). I looked at my child who was just 3 and looked at the aid that helped me pick things off the ground. I wanted to have a life with my son, go swimming, holidays, walks, all the things that other mothers did with their children.

I was now frightened (but did I stop eating?). I had been speaking to one member of the self-help group on the phone. She was bed ridden with obesity. She reckoned she weighed 36 stone. She had home helps, her children had been taken into care and she was diagnosed unfit to look after them (they were 12 and 15 years old). GP's had struck her off as she was too high a risk to keep on their records. She was unsuitable for obesity surgery as she was a smoker. Every door was shut for her. She frightened me as I thought she was my future if I did not get a grip. (I could not bear to be separated from my son, the f*****g food was not taking the love and joy of my life away.) I had hit rock bottom. I was defeated. I was f****d and I was very frightened. I went to see my GP who was exhausted with my constant visits. I asked my GP if he could refer me for surgery, which was called gastric stapling (this meant nothing to me, unheard of). I was in the pits and wanted a solution. I was to be referred and thought it would have taken a while.

CHAPTER 16
PREPARING FOR THE OPERATION

It was January 2000. Edward's dad's words still stuck in my head, "Who would screw you?" My name was down to be referred for surgery. I was still eating. James and I were doing OK. We had a good relationship (I never spoke much of my past demons; they were for the therapy rooms). James didn't drink or smoke. He was very creative and practical and stayed in the country. He introduced me to tranquillity and balance. We would stay in a lot and this would suit me, as I would try and not expose myself to social situations, as I knew people judged me by how I looked, and I couldn't stand pitiful looks or disgust. Fear of chairs and fitting into them didn't do much for me either and the public transport thing was an overwhelming ordeal, so I tried to avoid as much as possible.

My dad and Tricia hadn't seen Edward at this point in my life, and I intended to keep it that way. Edward had a full-time place at nursery and I had more time on my hands (a danger for a compulsive overeater – more eating time). I got a letter from the Western General Hospital, Edinburgh to attend and see a Dr. Ford in early February 2000. Things were moving.

Also at this time, I saw a course advertised for women who wanted to get back into work that accepted people with disabilities. There was nothing to lose in applying. James and I spoke of me going for the operation, but we didn't really know what it entailed. I had seen a result in my friend and I knew I wanted freedom from this restricted, trapped body (but I was frightened of being thin). James was supportive of me and respected my choice, but I could always sense an anxiety from him (but in this case couldn't put my finger on it). I cared a lot for James, he was not judgemental; he accepted me for who I was (with me constantly battling acceptance inside me). He showed me affection without neediness and was a very intelligent, insightful person who I respected. He never really shouted or got aggressive and sometimes I would test only the same balanced, calming approach to my crazy, needy behaviour. We got on well (I loved him). He took me away from my isolation that I had carried around with me for 30 years and I shared it with him. I allowed him into my dark world. I stopped going to the self-help group (I sensed some people there didn't agree with surgery. I didn't want to hear this). Also, I realised at this time that my phone friend from the group who was bedridden demanded so much of my time and energy. I kept thinking about her situation 24/7, I felt powerless over mine and powerless over her. Also, I think she was resentful I was being considered for surgery. I couldn't stand this negativity and energy draining and soon my door was slowly closing on her. I would not return calls or let the answering machine go on. I couldn't cope and had nothing to give. (I was still in the pits of food.) I had spoken to my sister about this operation that made big people thin. I was in the dark and so was she. We didn't know what this operation was; only that it was called gastric stapling.

My appointment with Dr. Ford came and I was weighed. I was just over 26 stone. I was told that I would have to demonstrate that I could lose weight before I was given the operation. I was told after the operation I would only be taking in soft foods and liquids and living on 600 calories a day. I would see a dietician (another die word) and get a one-off visit to a psychologist to see if I was mentally fit for this operation. I was to attend hospital for two weekly appointments where they would weigh me and monitor my weight to see if I was losing any. They also told me there was a bunch of people who met who had this operation and could talk to me about what to expect. I was willing to pass my phone number on and someone called Susan would be in touch.

I went home and decided that I would make soups, vegetable dishes and cut back and I would start going swimming. I had most days to swim and start changing my eating. It was difficult at first. I banned chocolate and biscuits from my cupboards and then no takeaways. I started to lose weight in the first two weeks. I lost about 7lbs. Then I started going swimming. (I still constantly thought of food). On the 14th of February 2000, James brought me a lovely card and gave me £100 to go and buy make-up. I felt OK. I went out and bought make-up and brought him some change back. I felt special and loved (but not totally comfortable with these feelings).

My divorce was in the final stages and Edward's dad had abandoned him apart from the odd visit if Edward was at his granny's.

It was round about this time I got an interview for the 'Women onto Work' course, which was going to be starting in April 2000. I went along for the interview in March, still sticking to my healthy eating plan (I hate the word 'diet') and doing some swimming. The 'Women onto Work' interviewers were very helpful and caring and gave me the time to speak and say why I wanted to go on this course that offered confidence building, job skills, creative stuff and fun stuff. They also informed me that it was a 3-day a week course that had disability access (which was important as stairs and I were no good). They also told me they covered all aspects of childcare. Edward would get collected from nursery by a registered childminder and cared for until I went to collect him. It sounded great but places were limited. I would be told in two weeks if I were offered a place. I would just have to wait and see (I wasn't blessed with patience).

It was mid March 2000 and I had lost over a stone on one of my swimming visits. I met a woman called Theresa (who is a dear friend). She had been cursed with obesity most of her adult life. She was 64 and still fighting with the scales. She told me she had her jaws wired and about all the prejudice she had encountered for being overweight. There was a woman with two grown sons in their 30's, who was a grandmother, a housewife, had been sole carer to her disabled husband for many years and went out and worked, and all her life she had given to obesity. It turned out she also attended Dr. Ford's clinic at the hospital, and also knew my sister, Maureen, from years ago. Theresa and I became firm friends.

Another time at swimming, I met a man called Bill who used to stay opposite my dad and Tricia in Bothwell Street. (My step-brothers called him 'gay Bill'.) He was always well spoken, polite and well dressed, never married. Theresa knew him as well. He said, "Oh, you're one of the Gallagher lassies, wee Sandra," (when was I ever wee, what he meant was he remembered me as a wee lassie). Bill spoke to me with sadness in his eyes and said, "What a terrible life you wee lassies had. Tricia and Pat were very cruel to you. You're better away from them, hen."

I always felt this victory that I had got away from them in many ways, but it was only physically because every time someone mentioned them, I felt that anger and rage and sadness at all the abuse, neglect, physical ridicule and beatings they gave me. I quickly dismissed my emotions, controlling them with food and inward anger (even though I was no longer in contact with them, I was still giving myself the same battering they gave me, only it was on my terms and conditions and that was with food).

I felt a bit of shame and exposed when Bill spoke about my past in front of Theresa. I was very good at hiding the past, even from me, and I felt annoyed and exposed, and skimmed over it with dry wit (a defence mechanism of mine). I said, "Oh, just leave the hillbillies to it". Theresa laughed.

Towards the end of March, I was told I had got offered a place on the 'Women onto Work' course. I was happy I had been accepted, and had not got a knock-back. I also had an appointment to see the hospital psychologist relating to the operation. The interview was pretty standard, routine questions, which I knew how to answer. I was asked if I was ready for this major operation, as ready as I was going to be. I also asked if there was any on-going psychological help before and after the operation. No was my answer, due to funding. (I was lucky; I still had my own therapist.) What were my inner fears about this operation? Well I was told being so morbidly obese the risk of death from anaesthetic were high, also complications during surgery (remember in 2000, gastric stapling was still pretty new in Britain and not that many people had had this operation). My worst demons were how would I cope with being accepted, how would I cope with being thin without this big coat of flesh that had kept me from me and people at bay. What would I do when I couldn't cope? I couldn't risk being put back into a psychiatric hospital and separated from my son, but I also couldn't stay where I was in a black hole of hell and a slave to food – unable to pick up a toy for my son or kneel on the floor with him. I spoke of some of these fears with my therapist and decided I would just have to practice patience and hope things worked out.

I also had James around me and he gave me stability and balance, so I felt supported. Maybe I was jumping the gun. I hadn't been accepted and I had some slip days. So I just had to wait. At the start of April 2000, I went back to get weighed. I was down to under 25 stone and Dr. Ford told me I was to be accepted for surgery. I met the surgeon who would perform the operation, Mr. McIntyre (a well respected surgeon). He was a nice man. He went into the medical stuff and a small diagram of what he would do. I confirmed like a lap dog shaking my head (I was not too bad at maintaining eye contact now. I had done my time with conversations and carpets). I didn't really understand what Mr. McIntyre was saying to me. He could have been speaking Russian as far as I was able to understand. I knew this man made big people thin or thinner, so I had him on a pedestal. What I had battled for 30 years, he had the solution to! It was now just a case of waiting for a date. I thought I was being tested on the patience game, but I was happy and relieved that I had been accepted for surgery. I had stopped contact via telephone with the bedridden member of the self-help group. I would send the odd letter or card, mostly through guilt and always hated it when she replied and expressed her misery and life sentence to her compulsion. On my next visit to hospital, I was told I was to go down to 800 calories a day. I was given replacement meal drinks. I was still eating pretty healthily and losing 2lbs a week. (I never weighed myself; household scales were no use to me. They only went to 19 stone.) I had lost about 21lbs in 9 – 10 weeks. The f*****g shakes / meal drinks were disgusting. I gave them a miss. I was on about 1,000 calories a day and was getting by. (I did have some slip / binge days, nothing to what I was used to.)

On my therapy sessions if the road got tough or too confrontational for me, I would sit and run into my mind (remember I had 30 years of playing roles and observing and being involved in crazy behaviour). If we spoke about things I wasn't ready to talk about, I would divert the conversation by covering up the emotion with intellect. I knew the therapy language and jargon, I had been in and out for 11 years now, read books, went to some workshops, so I educated myself with the talk (but doing the walk was a different story). So if the going got tough, denial mode and intellect would come in to save me. Sitting still but running away. Eventually, I did get round to speaking to my therapist about this. We decided we would try and be honest with each other and if we felt this defence mechanism was coming in, we would look at it. If the emotion was too raw or painful, we would address it differently, leave it or go back to it. I had choices. So this allowed me to work on myself without beating myself up. I couldn't afford to run back to the food at this stage in my life.

I started on my 'Women onto Work' course and met some great women who I formed friendships with. My life was OK (I was always afraid to admit that things were OK in case I sabotaged it or it was taken away from me). The course was good. It was nothing academic (I have dyslexia). It was giving you the gentle pace that you needed to see where your working life came from, where it was going, and working on the skills and inner stuff of self-esteem, confidence building, believing in yourself, looking at strengths and weaknesses and looking at work you could undertake with health problems / disability. (The course was for women with disabilities.) It was very well run and very well supported. I also went to a short course on parenting skills. I found it very helpful and informative for Edward and me. I learnt about reflective listening and communicating with Edward and other parents. I also decided to have reflexology weekly, as I had heard and read of the benefits.

Five weeks into the course, about the middle of May 2000, I got my date to go into hospital, June 14th 2000. I would be operated on the next day. I was very guarded about who I told about the operation. I was scared in case it failed and I felt a bit of a failure to be unable to do it on my own (but I knew myself I was beyond doing it myself, I was 16 stone overweight, the weight of 2 people). Not many people knew of the stick to help me pick things up or my inability to kneel or bend. They didn't know of the inability to wipe my own a**e. They knew I had a pretty face, if only I could lose weight. I was informed after the operation I would not be able to drive for a few weeks and be housebound for 4 weeks plus. (This didn't worry me, I was used to this.) I would have a scar going from my breast bone to my naval. I would be in intensive care for 2 – 3 days. I had to put practical wheels in motion with Edward. He would go to his granny's for a week and Blue with my sister. James, Julie and my sister would be at the hospital. Edward would come into see me on the Saturday / Sunday I was getting operated on.

On a Thursday, at the start of June, Blue had a visit to the vets. He was having terrible ear trouble (cocker spaniels were famous for it). They were bleeding badly this time and very smelly. He had this condition since he was a pup and he was now 9. It wasn't getting any better. This visit was to assess if they could operate on his ears. I took Edward to nursery and I went to the WOW course. At lunchtime I got a call on my mobile, there was no more they could do for Blue. I could bring him home if I wanted to and keep him on the drops and steroids, but he was in a lot of pain and his ears were all ulcerated. He would eventually have to get put to sleep. They said he could be given more sedation to keep him permanently sleeping and off to my mum and granny. I cried my eyes out that this wee guy had been with me through the last 9 years. He had never let me down and here I was going into hospital and had promised him big long walks and now he would never get them. F**k it! I found myself in a baker's shop, mascara down my eyes, eyeing up the cakes. I walked out. F**k this s**t. I didn't want to make this decision but I did know he was in pain as he couldn't stop scratching his ears and crying when he did. At one stage he had to get one of those lampshade things round his neck to stop him scratching.

I waited an hour and spoke to him in my car. I phoned the vet and let him go peacefully. They were all upset when I went to pick him up at 5.00pm. They knew him for years (it was the PDSA). I wanted to bury him in the garden when I picked Edward up and told him simply and gently. He cried his little eyes out. We buried him in the garden together and said a little prayer and put some daffodils over the soil. (It was important for me to tell Edward and not hide death from him. He deserved the truth.)

Just about this time James and I took Edward to the beach one day. He had his little bicycle and was going so fast down a hill he couldn't stop and went over a wall. I screamed. I couldn't f*****g run (my f****d body wouldn't allow it). James ran to him. We thought the hill was a big drop over the wall. Luckily, it was sloped and he had burst his nose and head. Blood was everywhere. I was gripped with fear. If the wall hadn't been sloped, it would have been fatal. James jumped the wall and Edward was screaming for Scotland. I felt it was all slow motion. I got him into the car and sped to the hospital. The hospital was busy. This was my worst fears coming back to haunt me. What if the doctors thought I did this? What if it was down in my records or Edward's that I had no bond with him as a baby and had a psychotic depression after he was born? What if? What if? My head was f*****g buzzing. I ate a bar of chocolate out of the vending machine without feeling it. I felt temporarily sedated. What if they took Edward away from me? I phoned his dad who hadn't seen him for six months. He didn't even visit him. James was trying to reassure me. I just wanted this sorted. Edward was drifting off to sleep and waking up crying. He got seen to and I was told that they would stitch his head in the morning. Edward still took a last bottle at night. I would go home and get it. I was back and forward to the hospital twice that night. They said I could sleep at the side of his bed on a camp bed. How the f**k could someone at 25 stone sleep in one of those beds? (Once again my excess flesh was in the way.) When I went home, I took two tranquilisers. It was the first time I had taken them for about a year (they were in my bathroom cabinet) and I ate some more food with them. I wasn't coping.

I got back to the hospital about 6am in the

morning. I could tell my laddie's lungs were working as he was screaming the f*****g ward down. There was a list of patients to go up for stitches. Needless to say, they took Edward first. He got home that day.

I went to the post-natal project (where I had belonged for two years). I knew you could drop in and see a counsellor. Edward was back to his usual self. I was a f*****g wreck with crazy thoughts. Edward saw their crèche, I saw their counsellor and after a few unsettled days of my demons and childhood, things calmed down. I took Edward to his granny's three days before I went into hospital, I knew he would be happy, safe and cared for. So I was secure with this arrangement and also scared of the hospital voices, the anaesthetic risks, surgery complications, f**k it, I was no longer a slave to fear.

On the Tuesday night, James and I had the last supper. It was quite an emotional night. I had a takeaway chicken curry with rice, chips, prawn crackers and a strawberry tart. James opened up a part of his life to me that night and I got freaked out. I thought he was telling me what he told me in case he never saw me again. It was heavy stuff. He told me his older brother, called Alexander, had hanged himself some years ago. This had happened in prison as he was going out with a single parent whose daughter had made an allegation about James' brother. James' brother was besotted with this woman and nobody ever found out the truth as Alexander hanged himself. James was in pain, the tears dripping onto his jeans. I comforted him and allowed him the time he needed. I was freaked out though at this timing. Maybe this was a confession, maybe he thought I would not see him again and wanted to off-load this burden to me. I was scared. Maybe I wouldn't get through this operation. I had discussed with my therapist that after the operation I was going to move away from Edinburgh. I didn't know where, but I wasn't going to stay where people knew me. I couldn't stand the shame of this failing or the praise of it succeeding. I wanted to get over this operation at my pace and transform without pressure. I didn't want to be in the limelight. I had given 30 years of isolation to this illness, so I was not setting myself up for failure.

I had met people through the hospital who had had this operation. They were all different shapes and sizes, ranging from 10 stone to 30 stone. We all met in the shopping centre for a coffee. Some had had the operation done and some were waiting. Some had maintained their weight and some spoke of hernias (no-one ever spoke of feelings or emotions). People spoke of how they kept the operation a secret from work colleagues. People spoke of what they could now wear and go to on holidays.

They spoke of how it was with what they ate now.

If they went to a restaurant, some could have a starter and a sweet. People spoke of still cooking for their families. It was all encouraging words and desperate people like me wanted what those people had. So why did I always have this niggling, nagging voice at the back of my head that something wasn't being addressed or spoken about. But I quickly dismissed this and didn't want to rock the boat and play the role of the outspoken spokeswoman. I didn't even know what I would be asking or seeking. I just put that baby thought to bed and got on with going into hospital for the new me.

CHAPTER 17

THE OPERATION AND TOILET BOWLS

We arrived at hospital the next day, Wednesday, James and I. I was given all the routine checks, blood pressure, and blood tests. I was also given a special electronic bed for after the operation that was specially ordered for morbidly obese patients. It came from down south. I felt embarrassed by this. James stayed as long as he could, and I phoned Edward. He was fine. I missed him and hoped I saw him again. My sister was coming in tomorrow. I knew she was still in touch with my dad and Tricia, but never once did she mention them to me or me to them.

My surgeon, Mr. McIntyre came up to see me. He referred to the operation as "vertical banded gastroplasty". (It sounded like a chicken pasty, only I could think of that one.) I never showed my fear to him. If I had been through stomach pumping in my crazy teenage years, I guessed I could handle this operation. Then the anaesthetist came up to see me. He was reassuring and told me he assisted Mr. McIntyre (I hoped in a positive way) and he had put people heavier than me under. I had broken sleep that night and as from midnight I was nil by mouth. It was a strange coincidence, but someone who ran a pub where my dad and Tricia drank was in with cyst problems. I never really spoke much about them, what positive conversation could I have about them.

I was told I would go to a side room when I came out of intensive care, and I would have morphine for the pain put into the back of my hand, it would be controlled. I was also told a follow-up procedure to the operation would be the cutting away of the excess skin that won't go away with the weight loss or exercise as an apron of skin hangs down from the stomach and also excess weight at the tops of arms, but this was a year or two down the line.

I was first to go down to theatre. I was shaking on that trolley; I was having a panic attack. I saw Mr. McIntyre with his operating gowns on. He looked different. He said, "Sandra, I will get you thin." (Why did I disbelieve him and feel a mixture of discomfort and relief with statement.) Nurses were speaking to me about where I lived, I hid behind humour, I said Leith area and I wanted to see it again.

The anaesthetist jagged my hand and told me to count back from 10. The next time I woke up I tried to get up. I was in intensive care and wanted a f*****g drink of water. I was crying and my sister had foam lollypop looking sticks, dabbing my lips with water. I just wanted the whole cup. I wasn't allowed. All this machinery was hooked up to me and nurses came in and addressed me by my full name, "Alexandria, are you OK? Are you comfortable?" All I wanted was water.

James was not allowed in but he stayed at the hospital all day, well into the night. It was now about 10 o'clock at night. Julie, my friend, had stayed into the night as well. I was sticking to the embarrassing specially ordered bed. It was so hot in intensive care and I was doped up. I kept going in and out of sleep, and I was having weird dreams. My sister left and I was meant to be in intensive care for another day. I was a fighter (my childhood gave me that strength). I wanted out. Mr. McIntyre came up to see me. I was doing OK. Everything went well. If all my checks were OK, blood pressure, pulse, etc. I got out at lunchtime and was put in my wee side room. I was f*****g sore. I was bandaged up. My wound was sore but the two morphine nurses came and told me how to administer morphine. I had a nice wee side room and I could drink water. I had some good luck cards in my bag (only a limited number of people knew I was having surgery). I had lavender oil and lemon oil in my bag. I had my walkman and pictures of my wee laddie and Blue.

I sat in my chair in my room, and for the first time in my life experienced gratitude about being alive. Nothing seemed that overpowering anymore. I was alive and I would see my wee laddie. I got a nurse to bring a phone to me. I spoke and heard his voice. I cried with relief and looked forward to seeing him. He was going to come in tomorrow with his granny. I got a small cup of tea and it went down OK. I dozed off and on in the chair. The morphine gave me nightmares. I wanted no more. (I had a strong tolerance to pain, my dear old father had seen to that with his beatings.) I took no more morphine (I knew I could not be a drug addict, a food addict, yes!).

James came into visit that afternoon and my sister and two friends. (My sister didn't like James, for no reason, she just didn't like him. I could tell by her body language and her ability to make him uncomfortable.) Julie came up to visit me that evening. I was still a bit doped up and tired. I just wanted to go home and be in my own surroundings, but I knew I would fight out of that chair and get home when all the visits were over. I phoned my wee laddie again. I just wanted to hear his voice. I was looking forward to seeing him tomorrow. My morphine thing was still in my hand, needled into the back of it. I didn't want or need it anymore. I would doze in the chair that night; it would be easier than getting in and out of bed. I took in some vitamin tablets with me as I had been taking them prior to the operation. I took one of those big f****g garlic capsules and a sip of water. After about 5 minutes, it felt like the f****r was stuck in my throat. It was very uncomfortable. After about an hour, I buzzed for a nurse. She came in quite quickly. I told her and showed her what I had taken. She told me that this was not advisable and said it would eventually go down. It did go down after about 8 hours; it felt like chronic heartburn alongside a feeling of choking. I didn't get much dozing that night. The Saturday after the operation, I was allowed another cup of tea in the morning, yippee! I drank half of it out of their blue plastic NHS patient cups. The two morphine givers (nurses) came into see me. I explained I didn't want anymore and wanted it out of my hand. They were trying to advise me against it. I would have to wait for the doctors' round; they were the only ones who could authorise it. The doctors came round and had the medical students with them and my core nurse gave them a run-down of how my blood pressure, etc., was going. Full smiles, I was doing well. (I was expected to stay in hospital a week.) I felt uncomfortable in my wound, not in pain. It was agreed I could come off the morphine. I wanted a shower and didn't want needles or wires in my way. A nurse came and helped me shower. I put on make-up and listened to my walkman. I was happy to be alive. Edward would be here in two hours.

I was looking forward to this all morning. Edward came with his granny bang on the start of visiting hours. I gave him a big kiss and cuddle (I loved him more than anything else in the world). He couldn't sit on my knee because of the wound and I couldn't lift him. He had brought me a get well card and flower. It was a hot day. He got bored after a while and went for a walk with his granny.

I lay on my bed. (I had got rid of that special embarrassing bed; I was on a normal hospital bed.) I hadn't looked down at my scar as it had a dressing and a bandage on it, but it was sore. I just wanted to get out of hospital. I didn't want to be sitting around a hospital. I wanted to go back to my own home. My surgeon, who had done the operation, informed me that he was the only one in the Lothians to do this operation and some other medics did not approve of it. He also told me we would be going into an obesity epidemic and that we were not so far behind America with lifestyle and eating trends. (I am starting to believe those words.)

I didn't want to keep in touch with the people I had met who had the operation. I honestly didn't feel any connection with them. Even to the point of being operated on, I suppressed my emotions (I knew my eating was emotional but I wasn't ready at that stage to look at the emotions). I had learnt a long time ago to mask these emotions and had learnt to deal with situations, feelings, thoughts and emotions in a very matter-of-fact way. I had to deny those emotions as they were too painful to confront without the proper help and guidance, and I was the one in control of them or them in control of me, that made me a compulsive overeater and sufferer of morbid obesity.

The intrusion and pain I felt physically and mentally from the operation was dealt with in a matter-of-fact way. I now realise at the ripe old age of 39, I have a delayed reaction to my emotions (I will explore this in further chapters). I got myself up and dressed on day 3 after the operation and put my make-up on and brushed myself down. (I blamed myself for being there, my fault, my mess, my dad's words, "You made your bed, lie in it".)

I was glad to be alive. I had small sips of juice, tea, and puree soup over my four day stay in hospital. I was ready to leave on the Monday. The doctors came round in the ward rounds and asked me how I was and were I OK. They asked if I had had a bowel movement yet! I said no, which I hadn't, but if this was a condition of staying, I said I would send them one through the post (laughter and humour another good guard for me). They laughed and allowed me home.

When I got home, I was empty but I was used to that familiar feeling by now. I opened my door to my mail, my divorce decree greeted me. I felt failure (but pushed it down). I missed Blue, my dog; he had been dead for about 3 – 4 weeks now. I made myself tea and looked at the food guide. I would have mashed potato with a few baked beans. I managed 4 – 5 teaspoons and felt very uncomfortable at the top of my throat. I just had a can of diet coke after that and a cuppa soup. I was given vitamin supplements away with me to take on a daily basis. I slept OK that night. I was in the house on my own; Edward was coming home in two days. I went to bed with the dressing still over my wound and I felt it very tender. I always tried to lie on my stomach, but this couldn't happen as it was too painful. I wouldn't be able to drive for about a month and would need help in washing as I didn't have a shower. On my second day in the house, I ate a little *Weetabix,* maybe half of one, and felt dreadful. I was starting to be sick. I wasn't feeling great. I went out for a walk and was being sick everywhere. There was nothing to bring up, just fluid. I felt frightened. I phoned the hospital who told me to drink a fizzy drink as this usually helps. I found this strange but it did not stay down. I had about 3 sips and was even sicker with a feeling of dreadful heartburn (like when you are pregnant).

About 7pm that night, I called my GP who sent a locum out. By this time I was throwing up blood. He was very concerned when he saw me. I felt frightened. He phoned the duty surgeon at the hospital and spoke to them. They wanted me to go back in. I said I would see how I was overnight and go in the morning if things hadn't settled. I was feeling very helpless, alone and weak. I went to bed with a sick bowl and woke every hour or so and was sick, which eventually went onto a black bile type sickness. The sickness lasted for 2½ days. I couldn't even keep water down. I was ready to be readmitted for dehydration, but it passed. In the first week I must have lost about 8lbs (but if you don't eat, you will lose weight). I felt weak, but kind of powerful as well that I was finally losing weight. I did not weigh myself as I could tell by my clothes. I had a follow-up appointment in 10 days.

Did I miss the food? Yes, I did. I used to think

about it 24 / 7, but I couldn't use it. I felt angry at not being able to fill the void, but also powerful and in control of losing weight (I wasn't, an artificial device inside me was). Did I ever think of that damaged little girl at that stage? No! …Too painful. Just as I had buried her with food, I masked her so a strong guard mask became even more powerful to protect her.

I eventually went back to my course and found it very difficult to fit in with social events, like going out for meals. As much as I was isolated, when I overate, I was now in the reverse in restaurants. I would have a cup of tea or a soft drink, no food. I couldn't cope with it. As much as people had stared at me eating when I could pre-op, I was now staring at them on the odd occasion when I thought I might manage some soup or something very light but I would spend half the time in the toilet throwing up violently. It was lonely and frightening, but I could handle it because on the other side of the scales, all my eating days were mostly done on my own or in secret or even as bad as in toilets. Once I went for my check up in the hospital, 2 – 3 weeks after the operation, I had lost 1½ stone. It was not very noticeable to other people, but it was to me. I had a daily diet of ½ a *Weetabix* with skimmed milk, low fat yoghurt, a cuppa soup, a packet of *Quavers* or *Wotsits* crisps, and that was it. I still cooked for Edward and if James was around, I would cook for him.

I decided I wanted to move away from Edinburgh,

I had decided that before the operation. I didn't want to be put on a pedestal by people who knew me in case I failed or they gave me praise or compliments. I felt this was a positive move to support me and not a runaway move.

CHAPTER 18

A NEW LIFE

I found a place 15 miles west of Edinburgh. It was a bungalow in its own grounds. My course had finished. My divorce was through. My body had been cut open and I was going onto a new chapter in my life. It was late summer 2000. Edward would go to a local nursery and go to a very small infant school for 2 years. The move was 15 miles closer to James and Edward's granny was 4 miles away, so I had some support. I just wanted to recover physically without any pressure from people who knew me (maybe I thought I was leaving the old me behind like the media and magazines tell us). Julie, my friend, was only 3 miles away. The move was semi-country and seemed positive.

I was still getting used to my very limited intake of food and also the powerfully tender scar that ran from my breast bone to my naval. It was August 2000 and I was about 2½ stone lighter and down to a size 20. It gave me great pleasure throwing all the f*****g tent clothes away. I would shop in charity shops for new clothes as I knew I would not be the same size for very long. As normal, a lot of the first few months of moving were taken up with dealing with schools, councils, decoration, practical things. By October / November 2000, the honeymoon period of the operation was kicking in with me. I was 4 stone lighter (I didn't weigh myself, the hospital did), and I was left with me and my emotions. Each day was getting darker and darker for me. I went to bed for a month. James and I were falling apart. I was changing physically and mentally (I think my body went into shutdown and my system was trying to cope with the impact of a very serious operation that had been performed on it 4 months earlier). It was in a state of adjustment, i.e., shock as it was being starved and so was my void and emotions. My only sanctuary was my bed. I hated myself for retreating to this method of survival, but I had nothing to support me. I felt really f****d, my head and heart was hungry; the artificial device inside me would not allow me to comfort it with my usual drug. I hated myself. I even felt I had abandoned me. All I could do was shut myself away, i.e., sleep, and I mean shut myself away, got up to the loo or to throw up. What an achievement. I had progressed from conversations with carpets to toilet bowls.

At this time, a friend who had come in and out of my life from my care days had just split up with his family and needed somewhere to stay, so Sean stayed in a room in the bungalow and helped me out greatly with Edward. Edward formed a great bond with Sean. His dad's visits were now nil and Sean filled up a part of Edward's life that I couldn't, like male stuff, football, outings, videos. I was not physically or mentally able. Sean helped me out as well (we never had anything more than friendship). I felt no threat from Sean, and I didn't need to be on guard from him, he was a very sensitive, gentle person that I needed in my life at a very low time. 5 months after the operation in November 2000, James and I were parting and I can honestly say it was more from my end I wanted to live (but did not know how); I wanted the grass is greener on the other side life; I wanted to go out; I wanted to socialise; I wanted all the things I hadn't had in the years of food. I was sabotaging James and I (and James was the only man I had ever cared for and loved, he accepted me when I was at my heaviest and I built up something special with him, but I was wanting to do all the things I thought other people were doing). James and I split up in November / December 2000. I never gave it any emotion, I just wanted to live. I started to go out on dates, men were starting to find me attractive (but I didn't). After all the years of people / men not accepting me, here they were, wanting to take me out, I didn't know how to act. But I did know dates were all I did. I still had deep rooted body image issues and I would not enter into anything physical / sexual. I was now 6 stone lighter and getting more acceptable to society. I was not in therapy and I was not on a high from losing weight. I can honestly say I was quite ill. On one of my dates out, I was invited out for a meal (tricky situation). I tried a starter that was small sliced mushrooms. I ate 1 sliced mushroom and 3 days later I was in my bed throwing up, followed by a 2 day hospital admission for dehydration. I felt very ill; I was hooked up to a drip and separated from my son. The medics didn't know much about the after effects of stomach stapling; it was a relatively new operation in Scotland. I was looking to them to get better and they were looking to me to give them feedback and knowledge of what was going on. I got out of hospital and had been frightened by that experience and thought I would never be back there. I hated being separated from Edward and he got very distressed about these sudden separations from me.

In January 2001, I decided I was confident enough to go back to college. I did a fast-track course in care and had seen it through by the summer of 2001. I had finished the course and my weight was down to 12 stone. I had follow up visits to my surgeon who referred me for plastic surgery on my stomach. As it had been so stretched, it would never go away with exercise (I was going to the gym twice a week). I was still having conversations with toilet bowls, nothing other than yoghurt, some soups, *Quaver* crisps, *Wotsits* crisps, *Weetabix,* mashed potato and gravy was all I could manage (very small portions). I was referred for the surgery, a tummy tuck, to cut away the excess flesh. I didn't know if I wanted it, but got put on the list.

Edward started school in August 2002. His head teacher had a weight problem and always used to ask me how I was losing all this weight (I wasn't, it was an artificial device). These are questions that I always wanted to avoid, I didn't want to speak openly about the operation, but I didn't want to hide it by lying. I would skim over it and make light jokes about it (humour mask aided me). People that knew me before and after the operation would have great feelings of envy towards me and sadly I felt this from my sister (remember I have a degree in picking up on people's feelings). These feelings would come out in social situations (that I still didn't feel comfortable in), and it always seemed to revolve around me. If men asked me out or showed me attention, my sister, or friend, Sandra, would demonstrate envy (and it's strange, because in all the time I maintained my weight at 69 / 70 Kg, I never had a relationship). I started to feel like my mum around men (something I never wanted to be). Men were not interested in me as a person; they were interested in the physical attraction. This made me feel even more hollow and empty. They didn't want me for who I was, but who was I? Even when my body was 26 stone or 10 stone, I always had a loyalty to me and my body that I would not have physical / sexual contact loosely. I didn't feel comfortable being around men I had no past experience or tools inside me to deal with these situations, so I avoided them (more isolation). I always used to look at media articles of people who had lost weight and saw the black and white picture of the big, huge, unhappy person and the glossy airbrushed picture of the size 10 women with a swimsuit on, laughing and smiling. I didn't feel like smiling. I felt lost in the world, lost without food and empty, all the things that the compulsion had robbed me of were still there. It took me a long time to look in a mirror and I still didn't like what I saw because I had addressed the exterior, so why didn't I feel complete, why didn't I feel like a smiling, colourful before and after picture. Because my head and heart was still hungry and I was physically depriving it and, once again, living in denial, people who got to know me had me on a pedestal. Medics shook my hand and said, "Well done". My surgeon lived up to his words, "I will get you thin". But I went to bed with me at night and I got up with me in the morning. I was empty, lonely, lost, but I felt I had to have gratitude. Don't get me wrong, I did to some extent. I could walk better and do lots more with my son (my knees will never come back due to wear and tear of morbid obesity). It was great being able to wear jeans and fashionable clothes and not get charged excessive prices for outsize clothes. But the stinking thinking doesn't go away (probably never leaves you). I used to look at chairs and wonder if I would fit into them. I had great problems with mirrors and it took me a long time to lie in a bath naked and confront my body.

Cooking for my child and other people was difficult. I had to sort out in my head portions and cook separately for me. People would walk past me in the street and not recognise me (sometimes I was grateful for this). I still thought about food, but in a different way. I thought about what I couldn't eat, and that was mostly everything. Did I feel deprived, I don't think so. I knew the physical pain I would be in if I did overeat, so I just knew where I stood with food. I felt once again I was in turmoil and battle with my body. Just like before at the other end, my dad versus me as a child, or society versus me as an unacceptable person (when I was morbidly obese). There was always a fight, a battle, a torture, no peace and no smiles.

CHAPTER 19

BYE, BYE FLESH

At the end of 2001, I had another four day stay in hospital. I was severely dehydrated and had been sick for three days prior to admission. My GP, who did not have much knowledge of stomach stapling, told me that I had a tummy upset. I told her that this was a bit more serious than a tummy upset. After day 3 I got admitted into hospital, dripped up and more separation from my son. I always knew at the end of these severe sickness bouts and hospital admissions it was like my stomach clearing itself out, not of food, because there was nothing in it, my weight was a steady 11½ stone, I was a size 12.

In January 2002, I went out with my friend, Julie, to celebrate my birthday. I had 3 drinks, spirits and diet coke. We drove back to West Lothian and got stopped by the police. I got breathalysed and my count was 52, I was 17 over what the legal limit was. (Later that year I lost my licence and got a conviction for drink driving.) I really wasn't much of a drinker. Alcohol frightened me due to the extent of what I had witnessed as a child, and what it turned my father into. I knew by losing my licence I was going to have to change my job as I was working in social care with adults with mental health problems and I required my car. Also, Edward was at an infant school that only went up to P3, and his school was 6 miles away from where I stayed. It wasn't an immediate problem about Edward as Sean still lived with us, thankfully, and would be able to transport Edward to and from school. I felt sad and let down in me that I had been so stupid to drive after drinking, but I knew I had to take responsibility. It would have been easy to blame the operation and the fact that I hadn't eaten much that day (or for the last year and a half), but I chose to take the alcohol.

In March of 2002, I got notification that I had been accepted for an abdominoplasty for excess abdominal skin (tummy tuck). I was wearing a pantie girdle for my stomach as it was not going away like the rest of my body, but it was OK with clothes on and I didn't plan on anyone in the immediate future seeing me with clothes off. I had only recently come to terms with that one myself over the past year. The surgeon that saw me at St. John's Hospital was a top specialist in plastic surgery and he took a photo of my stomach. Once again he praised me for my weight loss. The date for my tummy tuck was 1st May 2002. When I got to the hospital, the surgeon I had had the consultation with was not doing my operation, it was someone else who came up to meet me and explain the operation. He was a foreign doctor and very overweight. He spoke to me as a human being and asked me how I had managed to lose 15 stone. He told me he was so unhappy and just could not give up meat (I felt his pain). He told me people went to him to look good and he could perform this and they had him on a pedestal. (I knew exactly how he felt.) I trusted him because I knew he was a sufferer. He went on to explain the procedure of what he was going to do. He used a pen to outline across my stomach what he was going to cut. He said to me, "I pull you up, I pull you down", referring to my stomach. I had been pulled up and down all my life, one more time wouldn't matter! I decided I didn't want any more pain relief after this operation as the morphine had made me feel dreadful before. I took in lavender oils and alternative healing stuff. I never once thought or sought out advice or counselling before the tummy tuck and I have to say, it was the one operation that made me feel dreadful loss and utter sadness. When I woke up from the tummy tuck, I had been out cold for 10 hours. I had been given too much anaesthetic. I woke up at 10pm. I felt dreadful. I had this tubigrip around my stomach and it stopped at my breast bone. The pain was dreadful. I didn't feel my stomach. I felt empty and sad. I now understood how women must have felt when they lost a breast, my stomach was part of me and now it was cut away. I sniffed my lavender tissue and wiped away my tears.

The next morning, after a bad night's sleep and a lot of pain, I got up to the toilet and collapsed and banged my face off a wash-hand basin. My cheek was all bruised. I stayed in hospital for 5 days and the pain when they took the drain bottles out of me was horrific. I was told they had cut away about 3–

4lbs. I had a lot of stitches and a lot of pain. I will never, ever forget the loss of my stomach being cut away. If I could have reversed that choice, I would have I got back to my life, but this operation had scarred me. Eventually, when I took the tubing off, I saw the huge scar and a false stomach and they had made me a new navel. About one week after coming home from hospital, I started vomiting worse than I ever had. After 2 days, I phoned my surgeon who performed the stapling. He told me to come into hospital right away. They were frightened in case the staples had come undone and so did a part of me...But another part of me, at this point, didn't care. I just wanted this suffering to be over. Mr McIntyre, my surgeon, was organising for a dye to go through me, so they could see what was going on. I had been on a drip for 3 days and had nothing staying down for about 6 days. I was frightened of the results of the dye test. As sometimes, when other surgery is performed, it can interrupt the stomach stapling. When the results did come back, the stapling was fine, still intact. I was too physically ill to care after being in hospital for 5 days and on a drip. They couldn't find out what was causing the vomiting. This frightened me; they didn't know what was wrong. This is seriously when I was at my lowest point with the operation. Looking back, my body was probably in shock from the tummy tuck. I left hospital after 6 days. I was still being sick, this was the longest episode I had ever had, and honestly felt it wasn't going to stop when I got home. I weighed myself; I was just under 10 stone. I looked dreadful, all gaunt and drawn in round my face. Physically I could hardly move off my sofa. I was so weak. Luckily, Sean was still around to take care of Edward. I was a size 10 and it was summer 2002. My stomach now had 3 large scars on it, one from Edward, one from the stomach stapling and one from the tummy tuck. I was f****d. I was not enjoying this life, all the pain, was it ever going to be worth it? Eventually, after a further couple of days being sick, it all of a sudden stopped as quickly as it had come on. I must have stayed a size 10 for about a month. This was the worst time of my health. I was so thin, I didn't even have to wear a bra, my breasts had disappeared. I remember I was invited to a social occasion. I was standing in a night club and I wore a size 10 long, white dress. I always covered the tops of my arms with a shawl, as the excess flesh from them hung very loosely and I was very aware of it. I stood in that club and I was on my own with lots of people around me. All my life I wanted thinness (or so I thought), and I cannot put into words the loneliness, the disappointment, the hollow emptiness I felt. I had not one tool inside myself to support me. I was lost in the world, I was stumbling around with no direction, no path and very, very guarded. I had no faith in me. Other people did, but that was not enough for me. My interaction with men was dreadful and I just didn't have anything to hold on to. I felt cheated and robbed by myself. This solution didn't seem to be working for me, and I was finding it pretty difficult to hide behind my denial mask. Did I think by getting thin that my life would just slot into place. Maybe I did, all the years of magical thinking that helped me through the shipwreck of a childhood, the pain of being a teenager and sitting in psychiatric hospitals. Maybe all the dreams of wanting something I never experienced (thinness), why did it feel so flat, why did the f*****g demons keep coming back. Why was I unable to have a positive relationship with a man on any level? The more weight I lost, the more aggressive I became. The excess flesh had been a shield of protection. Now I had to replace it and still not let anyone into my world, my pain, the real pain, the real me (whoever that was). All the defects / traits that came with the compulsion were still there and emerging even more. The isolation was the worst.

6 – 8 weeks after my tummy tuck, I went back for a follow-up appointment. The pull up, pull down procedure had worked, so great it had been more pulled up. The excess flesh was pushed up and formed like an extra spare tyre. It was decided that I would be re-done. Another pull up, pull down. I thought it would have been another long wait. It didn't turn out to be that long a wait. It was July 2002 when I went for the follow-up appointment, so I assumed it would be another year. In September 2002, I decided that I would go away for a few days to a retreat in an abbey in the East of Scotland. I had been there before and I knew I had to take time out for me. Edward was going to his granny's to stay. I knew some heavy s**t was

coming up for me. I was going to court for my driving offence, I was going to have to move Edward's school and I was going to have more flesh cut away. On my visit to the abbey, some people from the West of Scotland were on a retreat from the self-help group I went to. I knew some of these people supported my friend who was bed-ridden with obesity. I asked one of the members how she was. They told me she had died at age 41. I felt like I had been punched in the gut. I felt sadness and fear. A mother of 2 children had been exploited by the media. Every door shut on her and sadly, and regretfully, even my door, and death, her final solution to this compulsion. I felt s**t. I shut myself away for a night and just felt numb and sad. The device inside me stopped me eating and I f*****g hated it. I wanted to eat, but I knew this was not possible. I wrote a letter to Linda, saying all the things I had wanted to say when she was alive and forgave myself for all the fear that had led me to shut the door on her. I spent the rest of my break in the abbey trying to focus on what was going on in my life and coming to terms with all the surgery and life change my body and mind had been through.

Even though at this stage in my life, I had a few opportunities to have a relationship with some men that found me attractive or wanted to pursue me, this was not an option for me. I knew I had nothing to give and was not ready on any level to be involved with anyone. I was still trying to come to terms with my new sliced body and my haunted mind. I knew it would have created more problems for me to be involved with anyone and it would have been so easy to take that option, but I owed it to myself to get well (in my head).

In October 2002, I got a driving ban, a fine and a short spell in prison for the driving offence. It tore me apart; I or my solicitor did not expect me to get put in prison. It was like a trip back to the past, more dysfunction, more aggression, a place of hell and sadness. It reminded me of my childhood all under one roof. I spent one week in prison and it was enough to put me back on anti-depressants for the next three months. The whole experience made me very traumatised and, once again, I never had much time to think as I got released on 29th October 2002 and on arriving home (Edward stayed with a friend and I kept the shame of prison from him), I had an appointment to go into hospital on 7th November 2002 to get my second tummy tuck done. Edward's birthday was on 8th November, so I was rushing around trying to deal with the separation of the week in prison I had and trying to make amends to me and him for the mistake I had made. Also, I was going to be separated from him again and especially I had to keep cheerful for his birthday. (His father had not given me any money for him in three years.) Edward had not seen his dad for the past two years (but was still in contact with his granny). Edward's school was 6 miles from my home. I had no car and no direct bus route. Why had I f****d up? Edward would stay with his granny and my friend while I was in hospital. I would be in for about 5 days and a plan for the next 4 weeks was put into place with the school to transport him there as I was unfit to drive due to my physical procedure. (I never told many people that I had lost my licence, I was too ashamed.)

CHAPTER 20

THE LAST OPERATION

On the 7th November 2002, I went back into hospital to get more flesh removed. I got Edward's care sorted out and his birthday gifts. I took a couple into hospital with me. As there were no beds in the surgical ward, I was put in the burns unit. You were not allowed in and out of the burns unit and visitors were not permitted. My worst fear and anxiety was I would not see my son on his birthday, but I was told that I would get moved to a surgical ward when a bed became available. The heat in the burns unit was horrific as no exposure is allowed in. I felt as if I was burning and dehydrating.

That spell in hospital gave me time to think. 10 days ago I was in prison; 10 days ago I started anti-depressants and here I was now, lying in hospital, waiting to be cut away again. (I did have a choice about the surgery, but the excess flesh was more visible with me a size 12 and bumps of flesh hanging down or up over waistbands.)

I was a steady 11 stone and my daily diet would consist of 1 *Weetabix* and skimmed milk (40 minutes to eat); 1 plain cracker; Lunch – soup, yoghurt; afternoon – banana (1 hour to eat); Tea – small portion of mashed potatoes, gravy and a small jelly. I had to devote a minimum time of 30 minutes to set aside to eat something, sometimes my tea would take an hour, and if, by chance, I chose the wrong thing, it was more meetings with toilet bowls with bouts of sickness.

This was my third surgical procedure in 18 months. My body was low and so was my mind. The hospital gave me time to think. I knew when I got out; I would have to deal with a new place for us to stay, with local transport and schools on tap. Where we lived just now was semi-rural. Once again, I was dealing with matter of fact, practical things, denial of what my body was going to go through, probably because I was s**t scared, scared of the pain from physical discomfort and pain from the loss of more of me being cut away. Why could I just not have been normal? Why did my body let me go to 26 stone? Why was it always me versus my body or my body versus me? Where would this internal battle stop? How much more did I have to take...? And through it all, I didn't feel the grass greener on the other side, and I didn't feel like the glossy babe that the media feeds us with. I felt hollow, empty, sad, a failure, but I reversed all these feelings to the outside world and played my role of success; false smiles, people pleasing. I took the pats on the back, but did I deserve them? I pretended and denied to myself that I was confident about this operation. I had been pulled up and down before, and I had survived a shipwreck of physical beatings from my dad. But deep in my small cut away stomach, I was a frightened little girl, and I really didn't know how to comfort me. I couldn't take my drug, so the only choice I had left was to put on a brave performance.

I went under the knife again, and when I woke up, I was informed that the operation had gone well. They had cut away 3 – 4lbs of flesh. I didn't want to hear the grim details; all I wanted was my laddie. It was his birthday and he would be 6 years old. All my planned hospital visits didn't frighten him too much, but the spontaneous ones did. He came up that night. I was still in the burns unit. I went out of the unit to see him, and wasn't allowed back in because of the rules and procedures of the unit. They found me a bed on another ward. I stayed in hospital for a further 4 days and this time took pain relief. I had one of those surgical tubigrips right under my breast and I didn't see the work until a few weeks down the line.

When I got home, I was around the house a lot. It was coming to the end of 2002, and wasn't I glad! Two major surgeries, a spell in prison, a lost licence and a three week stint in hospital for dehydration. I was glad to see the back of this year. Edward and I (oh, I forgot to mention our new family member, we rescued a cocker spaniel called Sally 6 months previously) and Sally spent Christmas 2002 together. We played football, went down to the beach and had a great time.

My operation had been a success. At my follow-up appointment in December 2002, the surgeon was pleased. I had two big aggressive scars running under my breasts to my back (I felt I had battered my body enough). I now have 5 scars, 4 from the operations for my morbid obesity and 1 from having Edward (oh, and one on my face due to the childhood neglect). (Me, I have more lines than British Rail, but I wish I had the correct line to me.)

I was happy to be home and so was Edward. Towards the end of 2002, I sat in my bedroom one night and just burst out crying. (Sean now had his own place in Edinburgh and came over to visit.) I looked at myself in the mirror. Who was I or what had I become and where was I going? (I still find mirrors uncomfortable.) Sean tried to comfort me and we spoke of how I felt. I didn't go into a long drawn out conversation, I just said how disappointed I felt and what a failure I had become. I think I was just getting a delayed impact of emotion to being in prison and the overhaul my body had been through. My weight was still a steady 11 stone.

Edward and I had great times. We went swimming and to the shows. We did things that the obesity had previously robbed us of. I didn't need the stick, but my knees and back were still restricted due to the wear and tear on my legs and knees. I was told I would always have the mobility restriction. I could not bend well or kneel. (I felt s**t about this, but had to learn to accept it and work round it.) I knew Edward didn't feel any shame about me and the obesity was at bay, it was in the past, it was cut away (but was it?). If I had sick bouts, I just had to be sick. They could last from 1 hour to 72 hours. Edward got used to me being sick. I told him, to the best of his understanding that it was caused by the operation I had on my stomach. Edward can't remember me being morbidly obese.

In early 2003, I got the chance to move back to Fife. It was ideal. The school was on my doorstep, a train link to Edinburgh and good public transport. I was going back to the same village I had set out married life with Edward's dad (and that I ran away from). This was a positive move. In early 2003, we moved back over to Fife and I got myself back to college to retrain. I got childcare sorted for Edward and I took a part-time job, 2 days a week, in Edinburgh.

I dressed well and off the peg. (I kept my one outsize purple skirt at the bottom of my wardrobe.) My weight stayed between 11 stone and 11½ stone. I still felt hollow and had no faith in me. In early 2003, I decided to go back to therapy. I could not continue with the head hunger and the feeling of not feeling complete. I knew I had a lot of footwork to do and not piss around. I needed things inside me to enable me to cope in the world and this is when I started to write this book in early 2003. New people I met never knew about the morbid obesity, but I did. Stinking thinking didn't go away. I would still look at chairs and wonder if I would fit in them. I would still pick bigger sized clothes. I still didn't interact well in social situations. When stress came into my life, I still wanted to eat. I was seeking tools inside me to be able to cope with life as it was now. The demons still came back into my dreams and in everyday life. Smells would remind me of my past or my behaviour or talk would remind me of my past. My emotional delay to situations and inability to express myself held me back. I knew if I opened the lid on the demons, the pain, the sadness, I would have to confront the damaged child and adult inside me, and I would not have my food drug to enable me to comfort the emotions. It was like a now or never situation and I felt I was ready for it.

So in early 2003, I started on this book and it opened a whole new can of worms for me. I went back to weekly therapy and I started taking honest steps to recovery for me. There were no highs and lows in my life, no dramas. The flesh had been cut away and the device inside me was allowing me to maintain my weight and I was a size 12 – 14. Each week I would go swimming and go to the gym. I would walk a lot as I didn't have a car. I tried to use the negative experience I had created with the car into a positive. In 2003, I was invited to a work party. On this night out, in the venue I went to, I bumped into my old social worker who I hadn't really been in touch with for 15 years. I had seen him in the passing. Gordon was very pleased to see me and we decided to keep in contact. He praised me for the weight I had lost. He knew some of my story and had seen me when I was in the pits of my obesity and compulsion. So he got to know the new me (even though I didn't). I had always looked up to Gordon as some sort of good, positive role model and he always listened and was someone who was honest and believed in me.

My sister, at this point, was in and out of my life. We were having major fall outs, just sister dramas, but when I found her too much to handle, I would back-track. I didn't tell her I had moved to Fife, I just saw her in the passing. I knew she was in distant contact with my dad and Tricia and I just didn't want to know. In late 2002, was the first time I had seen my dad and Tricia in probably 7 years, apart from the brief hospital visit. It was at a funeral and I was quite ill after my second tummy tuck. My uncle Frank, my dad's brother, had died, and I went to the funeral. I was the talk of the day, look at how ill I was. I wasn't the blob or fatso or fatty anymore. There was even talk from them that I might have Aids. This was the level of intelligence and empathy I expected from them. My dad was meant to be concerned about me, but never once did he come up to me at the funeral and ask how I was, or ask me for my phone number or if he could help me out (which I knew he wasn't capable of). I left that funeral hollow. I had now come to accept, at the age of 36, that I didn't need their approval or acceptance as I had worked through that they were incapable of giving anything. In many ways, I wished that I had not gone to the funeral as being around people, places, things that were bad for me made me feel hollow and negative. I was trying to simplify my life. I was reading a lot of self-help books and in touch with some people from my old self-help group. 2003 was quite an insightful year for me and a year of giving to me and spending quality time with my son. It was a good life, it was becoming simple and enjoyable, and I was learning to accept therapy for a period of 10 months. I didn't want to use it as a crutch or as a way of life. I had looked at some stuff I wanted to and just got on with daily living. Life was OK.

CHAPTER 21

ABBY-ROSE

In July 2003, I met someone called James, surprise, surprise! I went out with James for a date but realised that as he was a bit younger than me and we were from different worlds that I would not see him again and for the remainder of 2003 I didn't.

My body was coping a lot better with the operation and my weight being maintained and I had yearly appointments at the follow-up clinic with my surgeon who did the operation. He was pleased with my progress and was true to his word, he got me thin. My sick bouts were phasing out and I followed a simple 1,000 calorie intake diet daily. This is what it would be. I had progressed from the start of the operation from 600 calories a day to 1,000, but this was fine and I could eat a little more, but didn't over do it. I did weigh myself compulsively. From someone who had been terrified of scales, I would weigh myself about 3 or 4 times a week, and my weight could go up by 4lbs depending on my cycle. This would freak me out but I would always stay between 11 and 11½ stone.

Towards the end of 2003, I was friendly with a businessman who has always serviced my car for me over a period of 12 years. I would meet him for a drink or a chat. He was in an unhappy marriage, but I made it perfectly clear that I was only willing to offer friendship to him. I had met his wife briefly on a few occasions. I was able to have male company without intimate complications. Jimmy had known me when I was married at my heaviest and was very intrigued with how I had got to my weight. It was very complex to try and explain to people as sometimes I still hadn't grasped my own body loss / image or body truth. In December 2004, on Christmas Day, I spent it with Edward, Sean and Sally, my dog. Jimmy phoned me up at night having been drinking with his 7 year old son in the background and confessed his feelings for me. I told him that this was not appropriate and that it was not the right time to be saying these things in front of his son. (It made me sad that, once again, someone was giving me a mixed message through alcohol.) I decided to meet up with Jimmy a week later on a very awkward situation. My friend came along with me, and I spoke to Jimmy and said that nothing would ever happen between us. (I would never offer or come between a marriage) All I had to offer was friendship and I don't think this was enough for Jimmy. Over the course of the next few days, I really don't know how Jimmy had grasped my conversation with my position, but I had phone calls from his wife, angry and upset, thinking or assuming something had been going on with me and her husband. Obviously, Jimmy had seen my position as some sort of rejection, and wasn't capable of friendship. I wrote to Jimmy and his wife and made my position perfectly clear and put things to closure. I was very upset about the loss. It was my 37th birthday and I spent it crying. I didn't overeat, because I couldn't, and also this time was different, because I didn't want to. I dealt with the loss and pain and gave it the energy and thought it required and left it at that.

In late January 2004, I went out for a late birthday celebration with my friend, Julie. I bumped into James, who I went out with on the date back in July 2003. He took my number and I met up with him on 14th February 2004. I hadn't been physically involved with anyone for a long time. I had been doing a lot of work on body acceptance for me, looking at the loss of my former body and accepting my new body. I wasn't ready for sharing my body with anyone. I spent a whole night with James on 14th February. We just spoke and kissed. (Edward was at his granny's.) James arranged to meet me a week later. I went to meet his parents. (James was 13 years younger than me and I always felt uncomfortable with this.) I started seeing James about once a week. I could always feel protectiveness from him, but later realised it was a jealous obsession defect. In March I had arranged to meet him at a Social Club. By chance, I bumped into my sister. She was out with her new boyfriend. Some men were on a stag night and asked me and my sister to dance to a Robbie Williams song. It was harmless social interaction. James became aggressive and violent towards the men. I was disgusted and I left the club. James phoned me compulsively. His neediness was unbelievable. I had to get my landline number changed. After 2 weeks of mobile calls and letters to my home, I decided to go and meet him in a public place. He had lost weight and informed me he was on anti-depressants. I could not handle this neediness. I had had 3 or 4 dates with this guy and he was falling apart because of his inability to cope with social situations. I said I would meet him in a week or two. I really don't know why I agreed to that (maybe the compulsive caretaker in me). I met James in the middle of April and went out on 2 further dates with him. It just confirmed my insight. He could not cope in any social situation and was possessed with jealousy and control. I went away for a week's holiday with my friend and Edward. It was the end of April 2004, and on coming back I was meeting up with James and telling him that I didn't want to see him again. I knew I had nothing in common with him and he had nothing to offer me. I met up with him on 6th May 2004 and on the 7th May 2004, my daughter was conceived. I knew instantly, 2 weeks later my period was late and I thought I had a urine infection. I did a home pregnancy test. It was negative. The doctor gave me antibiotics. My period was still late. I did another test. It was positive. I did another test and took it to the doctor to confirm it was positive. I hadn't seen James since the 7th May, but I had spoken to him on the phone. When I got the doctor's result at the end of May, I foolishly told him I was pregnant, but I had also made it perfectly clear to me and him that us, as a couple, was going nowhere.

The pregnancy was a mistake and I was more worried about the implications of my physical health and the baby's with my restricted ability to absorb some foods. (James didn't know about my operation. We really didn't know much about each other.) After having a meeting with my doctor about my concerns about my health and the baby's, I was given reassurance. Also, a woman 120 miles away who had had stomach stapling had given birth to a healthy baby. I felt OK. I was booked in for a scan late July and I also had a yearly follow-up appointment at the clinic where my stomach stapling had been done.

James and I had no future and I made it perfectly clear to him that I and he (who hadn't even started) were over. I was going to do this alone. I was frightened and scared, but James and I were just a brief fling that had no future. He gave me a lot of mental grief from May to October 2004. I had no contact with him. Edward was happy. He was going to have a brother or sister. He was now 7½ and had adjusted into a happy, content, wee lad. (Termination was never an option for me.) I did have fears and anxiety about post-natal depression returning, but with proper communication, honesty and having lived through an episode of post-natal depression, no matter what I knew, I would come through it...But I was still frightened. My GP got me in touch with a psychiatrist, so we could set up a care plan and work together. I was not hostile to this happening, I was assured. I didn't have much support around me, it was Edward and I, and I wasn't in touch with my sister, but I felt OK. I had terrible cravings for black pudding and red pudding, which I really couldn't eat (due to operation). I had a craving for butter, which I could eat in small doses. The doctor who looked after me in my pregnancy was very helpful. Dr Tydeman wrote to the person who had performed the tummy tucks to see what had been done. (Apparently, there are different types and mesh hadn't been used, which was good.) My first scan was fine. Julie and Edward came with me. Edward was happy and we got a scan picture of the baby. Julie was supportive to me, and things were going OK. My college course was finished and I took part-time cleaning / supervisor job which was right on my doorstep. Edward's dad didn't pay for him and James was not in the picture. So I had to provide for Edward and I and a new baby. I had a few bad bouts of sickness that were not pregnancy related, but stomach operation stuff. I knew I would get over them but they were uncomfortable. My pregnancy went OK. I went for my check-up at the clinic for my stomach stapling and I was about 4 months pregnant. My weight was just under 12½ stone and everything was OK. I didn't really start to show that I was pregnant until I was about 6 months. At my second scan in September / October, you could find out the sex of the baby. I asked, but they couldn't see as the baby's legs were in an awkward position. I felt deflated and hormonal. I wanted to know, but just had to accept I wasn't meant to. My due date was 20th January 2005. I was booked in for an elective section (as history of Edward's birth). James got in touch in October and all I got from him was information all about him, anger and hostility towards me. I didn't need this. I told him I would contact him nearer the birth. (I regret telling him about the pregnancy.) I had supportive friends around me and Sean came over every weekend to help out with Edward, taking him to football, etc. My eating was OK and my weight seemed OK. The pregnancy seemed fine.

In November 2004, I had 3 meetings with my psychiatrist who knew about my previous psychiatric depression and hospital admission with Edward. We both decided that I would go on a mild anti-depressant in the middle of December 2004, a month before the baby was born. It was much better working with the psychiatrist and feeling I had choices. (There would be no damage to the baby as I was in the last trimester of my pregnancy.)

In November 2004, I also bumped into my sister and we kept in distant contact. Edward and I had a quiet Christmas together. We also made a tough decision, but a sensible one, to re-home our cocker spaniel, Sally. Sally went to a home in the country with 2 girls and loads of fields. Sally had always been terrified of men as she had been battered by one (I knew how she felt) before we rescued her, and the family we re-homed her to kept in touch and told us she goes everywhere with the man of the house, even to his job. She has such a good, strong bond with him, so I am glad she went to the right home and got her faith back in men.

In the new year of 2005, Edward and I had a viral cold infection. It was pretty miserable, but we were looking forward to the new baby coming.   didn't care about the sex of the baby, if it was a boy we were going to call it Ben or Adam; if it was a girl, we were going to call it Abby or Joy or Grace. Sean was going to stay with Edward for 3 days and his granny was going to take him for 2 days. Edward's granny spoke to me before I went into hospital and asked me how I could cope. She was referring back to Edward's birth. I got very guarded and said for one that I wasn't 26 stone anymore; two, I had brought Edward up single-handed for the past six years; three, I was a different person (and I was). I felt she was verbally criticising me and I gave back with verbal attack. I was frightened of all that past s**t coming back, but I had done the best I could and worked with all the people who were involved in my care plan and I did have support and insight to see me though, should the worst happen. I worked up to a week before going in to give birth and would go back very quickly. I couldn't afford not to work and my job wasn't demanding. Edward helped me pack my bag. It was quite formal. We packed it a week before the 19th January. I got a trapped nerve in my buttock and it was quite uncomfortable to walk and sleep, the baby was pressing down on the nerve. I had the room ready (I involved Edward with everything). We got the crib ready and all the baby clothes, the baby bath in the big bath, all the things a baby needs. I decided not to breast feed just in case things went wrong with my health, bottles were a better option. I would give the baby organic milk (which I took to hospital with me). I also put in some cleaning stuff. I wasn't being over the top, but I didn't want to get the MRSA bug again.

I had had some s****y nasty calls from James and some letters from him and his mother full of self-pity, angry, hostile words and a few nasty text messages. I didn't have the time or energy or want to feed into this dysfunctional behaviour. My main focus was my baby's health, my health and Edward's care. I was to be in hospital for 8pm on 19th January. Sean came over at teatime and I told him where everything was with regards to Edward and I watched Coronation Street, and then went in Sean's car to the hospital 10 minutes away. I had a purple maternity dress on and my make up and my bag with all my practical stuff inside. I got all my blood pressure, pulse, etc., taken and I was given a mild tranquiliser to help me sleep. Edward and Sean said their goodbyes (I could see tears in Edward's eyes) and I went into my bed. This time tomorrow night I would have another baby. A nurse came back with a doctor and I was informed that my blood was very low and I needed a blood transfusion. (Alarm bells started to ring in my head.) So the tranquiliser they gave me to help me rest served no purpose as with a blood transfusion you have to get your pulse and blood pressure taken every ½ hour or an hour to see you are not having a bad reaction to the blood. Just as I was getting into a sleep, I was woken up for all these checks and new nurses coming onto the morning shift asked if I got a good sleep!

I telephoned Edward that morning and told him I would be in touch with the school as soon as the baby was born. He would be the first to know.

I didn't want anybody at the birth with me. I felt it was too medical and I just wanted to do it on my own. People were at the end of a phone, should I need them. James' anger was unbelievable. He texted me the following message, "I hope you die you bitch. You're a failure. You can't give natural birth or breast feed". I replied by, "If you come anywhere near the hospital, I will get security to remove you". I didn't feel let down by these words. I understood his anger…. But it did confirm to me that, for once in my life, I had made the right choice and I wasn't going to allow myself to be a part of James' anger or unhappy life. I knew even before Abby was conceived that James and I were a non-starter. I just felt sad and confused that someone who had a family background and was so young could have so much bitterness and anger at other human beings (but I was not going to be in the firing line).

I was taken down to the delivery suite at 9am and this was it. I was put in a ward with a girl who had just given birth and looked in a lot of pain and the father was sitting rocking the baby as proud as punch. I started to feel frightened, this was it. I was told they were waiting on my blood results coming back from the lab. Why does 2 hours seem like 8? At 12pm I was told that my blood was quite low, but they would go ahead. I was wheeled in and 6 people in green gowns were around me. I was told what would be happening and was congratulated once again from the medics for my weight loss. I was told they would go back through Edward's scar to get the baby out. I was given an epidural, felt sick and a green shield was put in front of me. At 12.12pm on January 20th 2005, Abby-Rose was born. I didn't feel an instant bond. I felt relief that all had gone OK. I waited for her little cry and got stitched up.

CHAPTER 22

PARENTHOOD,
A NEW EXPERIENCE

Edward got his call at school at 1.30pm. He had a little sister. I went back to the maternity wing with my little baby who weighed 6lbs, 5ozs and slept. Edward came up after school with Sean and he was so excited. He kissed Abby and told her he was the boss. She then, at that very moment, had her first bowel movement. He was disgusted by this. I then asked him who the boss was. Maybe it was Abby! I felt on auto pilot but very tired. Edward went home with Sean at about 5pm. At 5.30pm I texted Abby's dad to tell him he had a daughter. He came to visit her. He was, or seemed to be, very ecstatic. I just didn't want to get involved. I gave him his time and really had nothing to say to him. On leaving, he said he would come back to visit. I didn't agree or disagree.

I was told that I needed another blood transfusion. I was very tired and my blood was still very low. I went back onto a maternity ward with screaming babies; it was very difficult to rest. I just wanted home.

The day after I gave birth to Abby, my psychiatrist came into see me. It was very difficult to see how I was as I was exhausted, but I seemed OK.

He said he would come and visit at home when I got home.

Abby's dad came back to the hospital for a further two visits.

Four days after giving birth, I felt all the old feelings with Edward's birth creeping back in. What if I hit Abby? What if I did something bad to her? What if I broke down? The nursing staff were very busy. All these thoughts going through my head, I was just exhausted. The maternity hospital was so busy and trying to sleep with screaming babies was a nightmare. Edward wanted me to come home. I wanted me to come home. My blood was not good and the medics were watching my wound. After a full week in hospital, Abby and I got released. Abby slept well in hospital (I think it was the intense heat). Whenever she woke, she would just cry for a little milk. She sounded like a little lamb. I telephoned my sister who was going to get my niece over to help me. Cherise, my niece was 15 and she was a great help. (This was all new to me, all the baby stuff. I hadn't done it with Edward.) Cherise stayed for 2 weeks. Edward was quite clingy and his nose was put out. He wasn't number one. I didn't push him aside. I involved him and he soon came round. I did have a touch of post-natal depression and sometimes the aggressive, obsessive thoughts would creep in. I knew I would get through it (if it really got that bad). Abby and I and Edward were trying to get into a routine. I was back at work part-time, two weeks after I had her, as I couldn't afford to take time off. I had a registered childminder put in to place and Abby went there 3 days a week from 4 weeks old. Abby was very unsettled on the organic milk. I quickly picked this up and switched to another type which suited her well.

Abby's dad was trying to give me a terrible time mentally by phoning my house and being angry and abusive. I just didn't have the time or energy to feed into his behaviour. It only made me stronger and confirmed that I had made the right choice not to have him around.

When Abby was 6 weeks old, I went to the post-natal self help group (which I had gone to with Edward). This was a type of group therapy and met once a week. I actually clashed with the therapist that ran the group and accepted this. I knew I wouldn't sit in something I wasn't comfortable with, so after 4 months I decided to leave. I sorted out individual counselling for myself at a counselling centre that a friend of mine who had been a compulsive overeater had recommended.

Between February 2005 and July 2005 I could feel my weight going up. I didn't weigh myself, but I could feel my clothes getting tight. I was now eating more, I was able to. I was not sleeping well and would get up through the night and would eat at the wrong times. People were starting to comment that I was putting on weight (this was my worst nightmare, and I felt I had no control).

In September I had a yearly appointment with the clinic that had seen me through the operation. I hadn't weighed myself in 9 months, so I knew I would get weighed in September.

Abby was now 8 months old and I was managing OK. I had a childminder three days a week. I had weekly support from Home Start, a charity which helps single parents. I was not taking anti-depressants (through choice) and I had put my name down on a list to see an individual counsellor.

James was still giving me the odd verbal phone call, and a couple of times I bumped into him. He was so full of anger and bitterness towards me. I was back working part-time (as Abby or Edward's dads were not supporting them). On August 28th 2005, Abby-Rose was being christened. I invited some of my family and my dad and Tricia (who I had seen briefly at a wedding in 2004, but my dad never spoke to me). My dad and Tricia never even had the civility to reply. This would have been my dad's last chance to see my children. I was so proud of them (maybe I wanted to show my dad what I had achieved and for him to share my joy, but he wasn't capable). The christening went well, and one of my aunts, my dad's sister, said, "Your father will have a lot of answering to do to your mother when she meets him again". This was two major celebrations in my life my dad had let me down on. (I honestly wasn't that affected. I had dealt with a lot of the rejection and abandonment from my father.)

One week later it was my sister's 40th birthday party. My dad and Tricia were also invited to that, but never appeared. Apparently, they were down at Tricia's daughter's child's christening which was in England.

September 2005 was my appointment with the clinic. I got weighed. I had put on 4½ stone in a year. I was referred to go for a barium meal, which would allow the medics to see if my stomach had opened. I would have to wait 4 – 6 weeks for the tests. I was now up 2 dress sizes and I wasn't compulsively eating, but I was consuming about 2,000 calories per day.

In September 2005 I had to get a medical with a DVLA doctor to get my driving licence back. In this medical, it was picked up that I had very severe anaemia, and quickly had to go on iron injections. (This would have explained my constant fatigue.) I had to get 2 / 3 injections per week into my hip. It was very painful and it caused severe bruising.

Round about this time, I was given an allocated space to see a private counsellor. What I wanted to address was my head hunger and my eating disorder. I met my counsellor, who was called Hilary. This time I didn't want to hide behind the jargon or speak about the weather. I was up front with myself and her from the start, so we got off on a positive footing.

At the end of October 2005, I had arranged to take Edward, Abby and Kevin (my sister's son) for a long weekend break on the Ayr coast (it was a family holiday park). Sean and his daughter came as well. We booked a caravan for 4 days. (I don't know why I chose that place as it reminded me of my childhood. This was where my dad and Tricia took us as kids.) For the first two days we were there it poured with rain, it was miserable. Sean and I decided that we would leave on the Sunday, a day early. I felt very low and flat, there the clocks were ready to go back that night, putting us into winter.

About 7.30pm on the Saturday night, I felt very edgy and just had this burning need to get home. Spontaneously, I said to Sean, "Let's go home now". It was 7.40pm at night. Nothing was going to stop me. We packed up the car very quickly and left just after 8pm. I phoned my sister to say I was coming home, but as a treat, I would take the kids to the cinema on the Sunday. We got home safely and all went to bed. On the Sunday my sister took Abby and Kevin, Edward and I went to the cinema. I felt very, very down and low, like a serious cloud of black depression was looming over me. On the cinema ending, my sister was supposed to meet me. She had sent along her boyfriend to tell me they were feeding Abby at his house, which was 10 minutes away. I followed him. I got to the house and my sister was sitting crying (I thought she and her boyfriend had just had another drama). She told me to sit down and told me dad was dead. He died at about 7.30pm last night (when I had the feeling to get home). My dad had died of a massive heart attack. I sat and cried with her.

CHAPTER 23
MY FATHER'S DEATH

I sat down and felt this was my worst ever situation I wanted to be in. (I always vowed I would never go to my dad's funeral.) We were to go over to Tricia's house. (I felt obligated, and now realise that this is no reason to do anything – if your heart isn't in it, don't do it.) I went into my dad and Tricia's home and it was like stepping back in time, the dysfunction was rife; the drink was free flow; there were about 40 strangers in the house, all boyfriends or girlfriends of Tricia's family; 3 pedigree boxer type dogs running around and a parrot in a cage by the window sitting saying, "Are you OK Pat?" (my dad's name) or "F**k off which people found amusing. The talk was all about what venue they would get for my dad's wake, how many people would be at the funeral and how good a guy my dad was. (Remember, this was all assisted by alcohol.) I felt I didn't belong there. I felt very uncomfortable. What was I doing there, sitting with a bunch of dysfunctional, needy children trapped in adult bodies? People, who had battered me, humiliated me, robbed me of my childhood, and had great envy of me breaking the cycle of dysfunction. I felt as if I was getting sucked back in. All the years of sitting with counsellors, doing some of the footwork, reading the books and going on to have my own functional family, would all this be washed or wiped away in a matter of hours? I felt angry with myself for being there and playing a role that I had to for these people. I was very confused. The strange thing is Tricia said two things to me that day on 30th October 2005. She and I ended up in the kitchen alone, and if ever I was to witness bitterness and doubt in someone, it was now. She said to me, "Sandra, I was with your dad for 32 years". I didn't know whether to say congratulations or commiserations. She also went on to say, "Sandra, you're all the woman you're going to be". (No thanks to her and her child abuse and neglect of me. What type of a woman did she know I was? Nil) Sometimes on the last thing she said words don't need to be exchanged, people sometimes know when a situation is or isn't going to happen. She said, "I thought you wouldn't come to your dad's funeral because of something my Aunt Ann had said". (This was Tricia at her best, always trying to blame other people for situations she had created.) We went back through to the living area; the room was filled with drunks and smoke. I just wanted out, it was just crazy. The phone was ringing every 2 minutes; the parrot swearing and people getting drunk. I was informed there was a place in the funeral car for me and Tricia would be in touch. I had no alcohol as I had an hour's journey home. I left after an hour.

On my way home in the car, my sister and I were once again skimming over the truth of the situation; we were talking s**t. I was trying to think nice thoughts of my dad, and all I could remember was the kickings from him; the way he addressed me as Blob or fatty. I felt so sad for me that I couldn't even bring up a pleasant picture of my father in my memory.

The next few days were dreadful. Demons of my past kept coming up. When I told people my dad had died, I said it very matter-of-fact and when they got awkward or started apologising and saying they were sorry, I said it didn't matter. (Once again, I became that battered morbidly obese child that would show no tears.) My sister was in a bad state. She was starting to speak about the sexual abuse. I couldn't cope. Edward was getting distressed by all this talk and dysfunctional grief and started to ask me questions about what my sister was talking about. (All the lengths I had gone to protect him from my childhood, my sister was exposing through her distress.) I felt angry with my father; even in death he was still causing distress, drama, and dysfunction.

I had asked Abby's dad to help out with her care. I told him my dad had died suddenly and could he mind Abby for a few hours. His answer was, "Because it suits you". I put the phone down, no words in the English vocabulary could reply to that statement. I was very torn about whether I should be going to my father's funeral. I kept going through in my mind who would I be crying for, me or my dad? (The answer is simple, me.)

I paid one more visit to Tricia's house, 3 days after

my dad's death. I took her some flowers. I was trying to be compassionate, but didn't feel it. When Maureen and I went back for our second visit, there were only about 20 people in the house. (Tricia surrounded herself with people as it was her way of running away) 3 days after my father's death. The topic of conversation was about me and who was Abby's dad. Obviously, my father's death was old news and my life seemed to be more interesting. I left after 45 minutes. I decided I was not going to be part of this puppet show. Maureen and I paid £45 each for a joint flower. Patrick, my father and Tricia's eldest son, was running the show.

On Thursday, 3rd November, I had tests for the state my stomach was in. I had a barium meal which I was told that as the liquid had went straight to my bowel, it looked like there was no restriction on my stomach, but I would have to go back to see my consultant in December. My sister met me and showed me my father's death announcement. In the paper it was worded the following way, "GALLAGHER, PATRICK. Suddenly at home on October 29, 2005, Pat, loving husband to Tricia, father to Patrick, Anthony, Frankie, Joseph, Margaret, Maureen and Sandra". Well, I am sure everyone knows in death announcements, the oldest children go by order; my sister was his firstborn and I his second. Margaret was not his natural daughter. Even in death, Tricia still couldn't stop her bitterness, her regret, her wickedness. This helped me in my choice not to go to the funeral. I was doing this for me, for my self respect. How could I sit in a religious room, full of people who had battered me, humiliated me, degraded me and sexually abused my sister? No, I had choices now; I could say goodbye to my father, my way, with dignity and self respect. My father lay in a funeral director's for another 6 days because Tricia couldn't get the venue booked for the day he was getting buried, so she left the poor man lying until the puppet show was complete. What I did for me was I dropped Tricia a brief note (that is what decent people do) and told her that I would not be at the funeral, it was my decision, and if she could respect that!

The one good thing, or positive thing, I had to support me was my counsellor and my friend Julie. Maureen was a mess but I had to put a boundary down for me. I told her that I wanted no more talk about them. My family were getting distressed and it was Edward's birthday on 8th November. I had to hold it together. Maureen knew I wasn't going to go to the funeral and she was having mega dramas, saying she was going one minute and not the next. It was her call, but I had made my decision. I was not going to be humiliated anymore. I was an adult now. I was not the poor, little girl that Tricia had power and control over. I had worked through the victim stuff a long time ago.

Abby's dad had seen my dad's death in the paper

and sent me inhumane text messages which I kept and got the Police to caution him.

My dad's funeral was 7th November. Some people sent me cards of sympathy. I wasn't grieving for the woman; I was grieving for the little girl who had to bury herself under food and lost a childhood. The woman in me was angry that Tricia was still the same old Tricia, the abuser, the controller, the manipulator. What I was angry with was that after 32 years, the disrespect she was still trying to give my mother's family. Decent people would have worded my dad's death differently and acknowledged my mother as being his former wife. Tricia never robbed me of saying goodbye with dignity to my father. When their puppet show of cars and tears were over, I went to my dad's grave and the soil was being put in, I put in a handmade floral flower for my mum and dad and photos of me, my wedding, my children and a letter to my dad as an adult. I said goodbye with my friend, Julie, at my side and went and had a cup of tea and met my sister and a couple of friends. My sister was drinking alcohol. On leaving after an hour, I advised her not to go near the wake, but I knew in my heart she would. I just wanted to get home to my kids. I felt a mixture of feelings driving home, which took an hour. I felt sad; I felt relief; I felt closure on something and I felt I did the best by me. It was no performance, no mask or act. It wasn't part of Tricia's puppet show. It was respectful to me, my father and my mother's living family and my mother.

On getting home, I got on with daily tasks. My childminder who was allocated to our family from a charity was coming and she would stay with Abby for 2 hours. About 6.30pm at night, my sister's drunken drama started. She was getting friends to phone me and she was screaming for my dad, she just wanted my dad (didn't we all in life?). It was like a 5 year old child having a tantrum. Maureen was going up to the wake to confront the guy that had sexually abused her (or so she stated). My phone was ringing non-stop with people around Maureen having great concerns for her safety and state of mind. I was glad I was 30 miles away, and I had an adult to speak to (childminder). Maureen's son at 12 who was very frightened wanted to come over and stay. I resented my sister for all the drama she was creating and a part of me, for just this once, wished she could behave like an adult (even though she was a damaged child). Her children, my children, me, were all being affected by her actions and behaviour and, once again, the good old alcohol. I knew the next day I was going to my counsellor, so I had support (and I was going, no matter what). I was trying to get my household back to normal and it was Edward's birthday. On Tuesday, 8th November, the day after my dad got buried, my sister had still not phoned, no-one could get a hold of her. There was nothing I could do. I sent Edward to school; Abby to the childminder and Kevin (my sister's son) was going to have to come with me. My heart went out to him. I was so angry at this point with my sister, I took Kevin for an ice-cream (and me, food = love) and I brought Edward's game boy. I had to see my counsellor, I had my 50 minute session, and when I got out, my sister rang my mobile, hung-over, unaware where Kevin had been all night. Apparently, she had gone up to the wake, screaming on my dad and made a scene. She sat and cuddled Tricia (one of my aunts gave me this information via a telephone call). My sister went on to inform me herself that she spoke to the person that had sexually abused her and the conversation was: my sister said, "I went in to see my dad at the funeral directors and told him Sandra wasn't lying all those years ago when she exposed you". His reply was, "Before your dad died, I told him I confessed to the abuse. And why do you want to bring it all out in the open as Tricia is still alive, do you want to hurt her?" My sister's reply, "Well, just wait until you bump into Sandra, wait and see what she will say to you". (Once again, my sister was trying to use me to do her footwork and play the role as I had always done as her compulsive caretaker). My reply to all of this was, "Maureen, your son is very upset and needs to be with you. Dad is dead and I don't want to hear anymore about these people. I will support you as I have said before down the proper legal channels, but I won't take these people on any other way and put my life, or my kid's life, in danger". I also reminded my sister that I had went and got her information on a sexual abuse support group (and she was going) and they would support and direct her in what choices she wanted to make. But now, for me, or her, wasn't the right time. I also expressed my anger and let down at the way my sister had abandoned everyone because she was on her own personal mission and everyone else was suffering as a result of her behaviour.

Over the next few weeks, I tried to get things back onto an even keel. Edward had reacted distressingly to my dad's death and all the conversation he heard. Sometimes, I would just be driving along and burst out crying, for who, I don't know, my dad, me, the lost years, the lost childhood, I don't know, but what I did know was that I was going back into my world of food...The warm, comforting friend and the ugly enemy. After I had said my peace to my sister, she became distant. I had to respect this for me and her. I got the odd drunken phone call from my dad's sister with false promises of coming to visit or meeting up. Surely at the ripe old age of 38 I was worth more than this. Nothing ever materialised out of these calls and I never, ever expected it to.

On the 8th December 2005 it was my mum's anniversary of her death. She had been dead for 32 years. I put a small piece in the paper for my mum and dad and me which read:

Sandra (Mearns) Gallagher 08/12/73
Former wife of the late Pat Gallagher
Nothing can stop the pass of fate

As amends are made at heaven's gate
Eternal peace and love mum & dad
Till we meet again
Your daughter, Sandra, grandchildren, Edward
and Abby-Rose.

I asked my sister if she wanted to be included and she said no, which was her choice. The verse I made up myself. This was my recognition to me, and from my children to their grandparents. It was my way of healing and putting an end to all the years of misery and distress.

Two weeks later I was at a Christmas night out with Julie. My dad and Tricia's oldest son, Patrick, attacked me from behind (that's the Gallagher style, nothing face on, violence solves everything). The attack was very feeble and was done in a room full of witnesses and CCTV. He also hit Julie. He was escorted out of the venue and charged. (I understand the role he felt he had to play and the manipulation that had been put upon him. I can just imagine the dysfunctional conversation, "Mum, I stabbed her to bits" or all the fabrication that went with the cowardly hero.) This was all for me speaking my thoughts and feelings (newspaper acknowledgement)…Poor, powerless Tricia. Strangely enough, the next day, my sister phoned me. I had a very strange feeling she was back in touch with them (but I honestly didn't care). She had a full-blown argument with me and made two statements, "Dad gave you life" ("Yes", was my reply "A life sentence") and she went on to say she regarded them as her family. My reply was, "Well, that's your choice. You can sail off into the sunset with them. I hope you get your happiness that you seek with them". ...But I was not being a part of them and conversations relating to them were not coming into mine or my children's lives. So I proposed that we did not see each other anymore and it was agreed (17th December 2005). I felt sad, loss and relief, but had decided that I wanted no more dysfunctional conversation or behaviour coming into my home.

CHAPTER 24
UNDERNEATH THE FLESH AND ME

On 28th December 2005, I attended my outpatients' appointment to get the verbal results of the barium meal to see if my stomach had opened and the answer to this was yes. (I knew it had). The cause of my stomach opening may have been caused by Abby-Rose and the section pulling and tugging to get her out. How did I feel hearing these words? …Panic. I had put on about 4½ stone in 11 months and I knew it didn't stop there for me. I was the only person in the Lothians to have a child after this operation and maybe it was constructive feedback to the medics that this operation is not suited to women of childbearing years. As Lothian was not doing anymore obesity surgery, only Glasgow or Aberdeen, my surgeon would write to my GP. She could see that I was in a state of panic. I started to ask about private operations, and the words she said to me left a powerful impact in my mind. She said, "Alexandria" (always got my full name from the medics) "You can do this yourself; you don't need an artificial device inside you to do it". It was the first time in 5 years since I had the operation that someone from the medical field had spoken to me with care and compassion.

As far back as I can remember this compulsion started with a packet of marshmallows when I was 4 years old. The impact my mother and father's divorce had on me was a big, black void and loss and I learned to fill it with food. The food chose me and I chose it. The death of my mother, the food was there, my close comfort and companion. The neglect and physical abuse and battering from my father, watching him getting drunk and smashed out of his mind, I got smashed out of my mind with the food, stoned and crazy, I hid my pain and shame under food, I hid me under food. People in the baker shops and in the biscuit shops showed me love and affection through stale end-of-the-day cakes, broken biscuits and chipped fruit. I looked into those people's eyes and they could see my pain and my suffering, but they would not rock the boat to the neglect or abuse, they wouldn't rescue me. So all I felt I was worth, or all that was on offer, was stale cakes and broken biscuits. I had a little girl's dreams before the compulsion took me away. I wanted to be a nurse, and I wanted to get married and have a husband and a swimming pool. Instead what I settled for was a life of nursing my dad, being a parent to him, and my swimming pool was a pool of food. I lost myself in the food, my friend, my comforter, my enemy, but by the age of 7 or 8, it was a way of life. It allowed me to survive the abuse and neglect; it robbed me of building friendships with my peers or to apply myself to any schoolwork or learning. If I didn't have food physically on me, I was constantly thinking of what stale cakes or broken biscuits I would get after school. Other children went home and got love and practical care. I had to give myself a quick injection of love from the cakes and biscuits and go home and face my abusers, then entertain them, then be a parent to them. My childhood survived through food.

As a morbidly obese child in the early to mid 70's, I was in the minority. I was different to my other peers and I would be unable to join in some things, e.g., sports or physical activity. I would also be called names by other children, like fatty or fatso, and I knew how to handle this, the way I had been shown, with aggression. I wasn't over the top aggressive, but I could handle myself. I had to, to enable me to survive my home life and school was a refuge. The things I did to enable me to feed my habit, like steal or befriend people, I hated. I hated it so much, but it was desperation, it was survival. I knew it was wrong, even as an eight year old and this made it worse. This is one side of the compulsion that really ate away at me. There were no boundaries or rules. Needs must and, at that stage, I needed food (and in some ways, I thought food needed me).

Thirty five years I have given to this compulsion. I have been round the whole system and back again. On one hand, I am an expert in the field, and on the other hand, I am very much in the dark. Intellect of this compulsion will not stop me actively doing it. Cutting away the FAT will not stop me doing it. Artificial devices will not stop me doing it; slimming clubs and acupuncture will not stop me doing it. I am separate from the compulsion and the obesity is a symptom of the head and heart hunger. I have never, ever experienced real hunger or real fullness in all my life. One bite is too many and fifty is not enough. Compulsive overeating is still not recognised in the medical field; anorexia and bulimia is; compulsive overeating, no, we are still in the dark about it. It is just as dangerous as any other eating disorder, but is the solution to put artificial devices or cut away the fat. I don't believe so. People may be suffering head hunger and heart hunger (when I say heart, I mean, belief, spiritual, faith). The government is now considering stomach stapling for children as young as 12 years old. Treating the symptom, not the cause (and each cause is individual). Is it right for a 12 / 14 year old to have deep, intrusive, physical surgery? An intrusive operation that may allow the body to go to an acceptable size and follow-up procedures of more surgery to put right the excess skin and not address the cause. It is only treating the physical symptom, and for me, back in 2000, when I had my operation, I wanted a solution. I wanted my life back and, to some degree, I did in the physical sense. But because an artificial device goes inside you, it does not take away the emotional hunger and pain. It does not take away years of stinking thinking, of looking at chairs and wondering if you can fit in them. Compulsive overeating is cunning. The sad thing about this compulsion is you need to eat to live and sometimes, when you are in the pits of the compulsion, all you do is live to eat. I have been cut away but not cut off from my feelings and thoughts. The word FAT, a small word with a big meaning, means, for me, a compulsive eater, feelings and thoughts. It has always been that for me, that 4 year old little girl who had to eat the whole packet of marshmallows, experienced her first ever FAT experience, and continued for the next 35 years. When I went for surgery at 33 years old, I felt I didn't have a choice. Death was facing me head on. 28 stone, my heaviest. No boundaries, rules or regulations with this compulsion. Next year I could be 40 stone or 10 stone. Some people commented to me that if you can't diet yourself, you're a failure. (I was, and always will be, beyond diets.) I felt I had no choice. People who get surgery for morbid obesity are very brave people to put your body into intensive care (in my case, my compulsion put me there) and throw up for 2 – 3 years and have 4 hospital admissions. They are not a failure. Obesity surgery is a big business, £8 - £10,000 for an operation. To treat symptoms, not the cause, unless there is any medical reason for someone being obese, only they will know the reasons why they feel the need to be big and to keep feeding the head and heart.

My eating disorder is threefold. In nature it is physical, emotional and spiritual. I am not someone who just enjoys food. I don't know when to start eating and I don't know where to stop. The compulsion has been very lonely and isolating. I have lived in a world of denial, fear, sadness, physical and emotional pain for many years. The masks I have created in order to protect myself (even from me) and the behaviour I have indulged in or demonstrated whilst being high / low on food was once again, a defect of the illness. The risks I have taken to eat, driving to shops in the middle of the night, all to fuel the compulsion. Driving along and stuffing the food in my face, with no regard for my life or the lives of others, eating my children's sweets or stealing food that doesn't belong to me. The humiliation and guilt I have put myself through is immense. I have given 150% to this compulsion. I have denied jobs, holidays, people, relationships and most of me. Underneath all my flesh and my character defects I am shy, caring, sensitive and loving person. My masks only protect me from the observer; deep down they don't protect me from me. I go to bed with me and I get up with me. The food, the abuse, the neglect, the injected dysfunction, all made me into the person I had become. I went to the slimming clubs. I went to the medics looking for a solution or an answer to how or why I had become what I saw, a mass of flesh. On one hand, it was invisible to me, on the other hand, rejected by me, rejected by society. As I had spent 30 plus years in a fog of denial, when all the weight was cut away and controlled by a device, I was left with an even hollower, empty void. I did not know how to interact with others; how to have relationships; how to live / survive with or without food. So as much as I was lost in the world when I was morbidly obese, I had no tools inside me to live or cope in the thin world. I felt even more betrayed. But deep down inside, I knew it was always more than cutting the flesh away, but that was what the only treatment was, cutting away the flesh, that was all that was on offer, just like the stale cakes and broken biscuits when I was 7. I felt I didn't have a choice, so I went and I got the flesh cut away. In the finishing of this chapter, I have written some poems over the years that explain what it was like and helped me to understand it when the world couldn't.

LOST YEARS

All the years of filling myself with food,
Trying to make me feel wanted and good,
I will never have the answers why this compulsion came to me,
As all my life I have run from it and tried to be free,
The pain it has given my body and head,
The cause may have been loss or a wrong word said,
But all I know it is something that had to be constantly fed,
The sad thing about this one is we have to eat to live,
But I realise now that my self-will has to give,
As I want to see and feel the joy and love others have had,
And not run and hide in food, always feeling bad.

THE OPERATION

They can cut away the fat and get the desired effect we seek,
As long as the feelings are shut in and we don't let them leak,
People can say we look well, and we can now play our part and look and be acceptable,
But deep inside our head and feelings are we stable,
We still look at doors and chairs with fear,
Because our compulsive thinking has not been able to clear,
No tools inside us to equip us with the person we have become,
We have paid the price for this operation and maybe even been stung,
The medics can only go on what they know,
But we are the ones that have performed the show,
There's no earth solution to being overweight,
Who knows we might get the answer we seek at heaven's gate.

TO MY DAD

I wanted your arms to pick me up, and protect me
and give me feelings of love and joy,
But the little girl inside me, bit by bit, you set out to
destroy,
You robbed me of my dolls and teddy bears,
Left alone to get on with it, knowing no one cared,
I became your parent and put my life on hold,
Always having to be growing up and acting old,
I wore many masks for you to hide away my fear,
Kicked and punched and humiliated year after
year,
I ran to food to make me big, to love me and hold
it together within,
And all my adult life I was rejected all over again
for not being thin,
I never got the amends from you as you were
taken to your grave,
And now the fight inside me has stopped, there is
nothing left for you and me to save,
I feel sad you never saw the woman I had become
or the grandchildren I bore,
But when we meet again dad, please be waiting at
heaven's door.

From your daughter, Sandra

MY LIFE IN FOOD

Always running to hide in food,
To numb my feelings and alter my mood,
Using the food to hide the real me,
As fear stops people getting too close to look in and see,
The sugar highs and lows and feeding the empty hole,
For all the emotions and feelings that those people stole,
The slow pain of the comforter eating,
Never giving me an answer to what it is I am seeking,
It could be love or acceptance of who I have become,
But in this compulsion it does not equal like some simple sum,
The emptiness and isolation this illness creates,
I don't know if there will ever be a solution for 33 years I have had to wait,
I just hope that the food doesn't hold the key to my fate!

CHAPTER 25
MAKING AMENDS

After 30 plus years of battering my body and head with food, the first person I had to make amends to, was me (and sometimes this is easier said than done). But it is important that I continue doing this to myself. For 30 plus years, as much as my father physically and mentally battered me as a child, I continued it all through my adult life, filling my thoughts and feelings with food. My body was getting bigger, my inability to bend or kneel, it was physical punishment. Making amends to me doesn't just fit like a slipper. It has to take form on a daily basis and means being kind to myself, looking after myself by doing things like going swimming with my children, going for a walk, eating sensible food, forming friendships with people, trusting myself and people, sharing my emotions with my counsellor, allowing myself to cry if it is appropriate and feeling no shame, playing with my children and having fun with them and recognising everything I have always sought. My morbidly obese, f****d, fatso, fatty, blob (all the names given to me). Thank you dear body, you allowed me to have two beautiful children and allowed me to be a family, something I always sought. You didn't give up or let me down. Every day, when I have a bath or look in a mirror, and I am able to do that now, I see the scars, the scars of the 3 operations. But I accept that this is where my compulsion took me. I don't fight or deny that part of my life. I don't hide away from it; the scars meet me every day. I accept. I also don't promote physical procedures. It is an individual choice, but it's certainly not a solution. All the behaviours and dramas I fed into, I have to take responsibility for. The stealing I deeply regret. I have a criminal record and the justice system dealt with me. I knew it was wrong and each day I put loose change in a jar and give to two charities each year. I also donate monthly to two charities (one being a children's charity). This is the correct thing for me to do. I also do voluntary work and give back some service. I constantly seek and invite balance and simplicity into my life and I have to stay away from people, places and things that are bad for me. Each week I see a counsellor and work on these areas in my life and the food takes care of itself. It is not easy and needs constant work and commitment, but this is making amends to me, this is taking care of me. As a single parent, I am mother and father to my children. I provide the food and there is extra pressure on me to be a good role model. We sit and eat meals at a table as a family. We don't make big issues about food and, if I am actively in the compulsion (and some days I still am or will be), I try and avoid doing this in front of my children. I remember my mum's bulimia and water sipping days. She was my role model and I remember her anxiety and despair and torture around food. I will go to all lengths for my children not to see my compulsion when I am in the pits of despair. One blessing is Edward can't really remember me being 28 stone. He has seen pictures and once asked, "Who was that, mum?" I am not ashamed of that 28 stone person. I am honest with my son and tell him I was very unhappy and we have spoken about the operation I went for. He knows a little about my unhappy childhood and he knows why I never took him to see my father. I have given him enough information and respect for his age and what he could cope with. My dysfunctional abusive childhood gave me the insight and awareness to be a good parent to my children. I give them morals, values, boundaries, love and care; all the things that my father should have given to me. Have I forgiven my father? I am trying to and willing to. I always dreamed or fantasised that I would get huge, big, remorseful amends from my father and one day get the confrontation with him that I so much sought and deserved, but that takes two adults to make that happen and my dad wasn't an adult. He was an unhappy boy trapped in a man's body, and, as a result of his unhappiness, he made most people who came into contact with him miserable and unhappy. Sometimes, I get peace and serenity when I think whatever he could not do for himself or me on earth; he may be able to do wherever his spirit has gone. As for Tricia, Tricia is still on earth and I am living proof that Tricia is a child abuser and a person who contributed a lot of physical and mental abuse to me. I don't think of Tricia a lot, I know as an adult what Tricia is, a manipulative, controlling, angry, unhappy person. Even on my dad's death, she still tried to take away my spirit and my being. She tried for all those years when I was a powerless little child. Also, my name was Sandra, named after my mother, so this was more salt in her wounds. I would have been quite willing to meet Tricia at one point in my life and tell her exactly what I thought, but it really would not have done me any good and, once again, that takes two adults to enter into a meeting like that and, having observed, and actively received, years of her crazy behaviour, I am qualified to say that she was not worthy or capable of my adult time.

The statement she made to me on my dad's death, "You're all the woman you're going to be". Yes, I am, with no proper input or help from her. Maybe she should have reflected that statement back to her. What an achievement in life; neglect, cruelty and abuse to a dead woman's kids. The saddest thing is that she was a mother to children herself! I wish Tricia no bad and no good. She means very little to me (and this is making amends to me). In 1997, after my granny died, I wrote an eight page letter to my aunt and uncle who had nursed my mum on her death. I told them what it was like for me and we had a good few meetings and spoke about our feelings and thoughts. The rest of my mum's family I don't see.

My sister and I; It has taken me a long time to get some understanding of mine and my sister's relationship. The two little china dolls that my mum cherished got lost and destroyed in the years of abuse and neglect from our years with my dad and Tricia. It was survival, no regard for each other; my sister played her role of the victim and me the survivor. To this day, when we are in contact with each other, we still play these roles. For me, I am tired and don't want or need to play the roles anymore, because when I do, I go back to my masks of people-pleasing, false strength, neglect of my own needs and that dysfunctional feeling of my dad and Tricia having power over me. I am then led back to my friend, my strength, my love, food, and I can't do it anymore. After my father's death, a strong observation came to my eyes, and this was that there are no winners or losers in abusive upbringing; all there is, is living proof of that.

I don't see my sister and have not for 8 months, but I hope she gets peace and happiness from life that she deserves. I respect the choice the two of us have made and that is to go on different paths and it is not so bad, it's OK.

On my divorce with Edward's dad, I wrote him a letter (it is in my drawer). I was so desperate for someone to love me when I met Edward's dad, but if you have not received that in life, or love yourself, or even care for yourself, no one else can give you that. Edward's dad did try, but I sabotaged any affection I was ever shown. I couldn't give, or receive; I had no insight or awareness into love or affection. All my life I was starved of it, so I used food and allowed people to hurt me and I hurt them. I make amends to myself for that behaviour. I didn't know how to go about any different behaviour and I was not ready to allow anyone in my life. All that was there was food. It had served me for all those years, so there was no room for a third person. It was me and food and a big, empty, hollow void.

In 1997, I reported the abuse and neglect that happened in the local authority care to the police and there was a huge investigation. Julie and I went through a two year period of interviews, meetings and I had counselling. The positive outcome was a children's charter was set up for children in care, and at the disciplinary hearing, the staff that were involved or left working for the authority either got demoted or suspended or moved out of working with vulnerable people. I also note, with great relief that a children's charter is in place for children now. I look down the list and see mostly everything on that list, I experienced firsthand from my dad and Tricia. I feel sad that there was none of this charter to save me when I was young and robbed me of my childhood.

I also forgave the teachers and the food givers and the neighbours and my mum's family for not rescuing us. For whatever reasons, they chose not to, they showed care and concern and affection through food. I am sure if they had known where those stale cakes and broken biscuits took me to, they may have demonstrated their care in another way.

Amends and forgiveness allows me freedom. It is something that continues on a daily basis for me. There are many people out there who could have, or should have, made amends to me. But I have done my part and will continue to do so and some people have been adult enough and respected me enough to make amends. Amends and forgiveness has required a great deal of honesty from me, something I thought I would never be able to do, to give it or receive it, and it feels OK, it feels right for me, and it enables me to have freedom from my compulsion.

The situation I have always struggled to come to terms with is the disability the compulsion has left me with, the inability to bend and kneel. When I got down to 11 stone with the assistance of the artificial device in me, I always had magical thinking that I would be able to bend and kneel. Sadly, this didn't happen. I have mobility restriction, due to wear and tear of my knees and back, due to years of food abuse and morbid obesity. I don't fight this anymore. I work on acceptance of this condition and I don't beat myself up. It happened and nothing will change it.

CHAPTER 26
NO MAGICAL RAINBOWS OR SOLUTIONS

I would have liked to end this book by stating this is my solution to compulsive overeating and morbid obesity. But this is an honest admittance of 35 years of my life. Yes, I am an expert in this illness and also in the dark. My experience is there is no solution to compulsive overeating or morbid obesity. There are diet clubs, there are self-help books, groups, herbal remedies, clothing remedies, needle remedies, surgical procedures, but there is no solution, no magical rainbows, no wonder cures. What I have had from compulsive eating is daily / weekly / monthly reprieves – freedom, and the methods I used for my head and heart hunger worked on a daily basis for me.

On January 2006, after a meeting with my GP, and weighing 113kgs, I was referred to a surgeon in Glasgow who performs obesity surgery as my previous operation had opened up after I had my daughter and I had maintained a 3 year weight loss of 16 stone (my weight stayed at 11stone) with an artificial device in me. I came away from the surgery feeling good, feeling happy and I had some food to celebrate. I was getting considered for more surgery. Things wouldn't get unliveable again. More knives and devices would sort me out. Then a day later, I sat down and cried. I cried my eyes out. After 6 years of hospitals, being cut away, hospital admissions for vomiting and dehydration, separation from my children, could I really put my body, myself and my children through all that again, the answer was with me and always had been no. No more knives, no more devices, no more mental and physical pain and torture, no more. I was living, or had been living, a pattern very similar to my childhood, still getting battered emotionally and physically. No more, enough was enough. I had a choice, not a solution. So I decided that I would set out a life change that suited me as an individual, a plan that I could follow and, if I slipped back into the compulsion, I would not beat myself up. I decided that I would exercise twice a week for 1 hour each session on my own. I would also involve my children in a walk or a swim or cycle on a daily basis. I would continue with weekly appointments with my counsellor and speak honestly and feel the emotions and thoughts. I would visit a supermarket once a fortnight to shop for the food we required as a family. I would not bring into my home foods that distressed me. I would set aside time for me each morning and do a daily reading from my fellow sufferers' book. I would keep a diary daily of my feelings and thoughts (not my food). I would not weigh myself, but would have awareness from my diary and my clothes what my eating was like. I would do something for me each day that would boost my confidence and self esteem and this could be changing my hairstyle or wearing a nice piece of jewellery or scarf. I would strive to keep my life simple and balanced, and avoid people, places and things that were bad for me. I would listen to my inner self and see what my needs were and try to meet them. I would cook food which I wanted and felt was healthy for me and put it into acceptable portions and freeze some for the coming week. If I go to a social occasion, I will carry light food of my own with me and if anyone confronts me about why I am doing this, I will not say I am dieting, which is the truth, I will say that I am following a special eating plan and leave it at that. I am not willing or wanting to fight with food anymore, it will always win the battle because I accept that I have no power or control over it. Each day when I have a reprieve / recovery from the illness, I am grateful. Some days, new revelations and awareness comes to me and I am open to this.

I would love to take a magical pill and this compulsion to be removed. But I would still have to do the head and heart work. I would still be left with me. I would rather just do the talk than so the walk. But the walk really does not frighten me anymore. I have set up a plan, a lifestyle plan that suits me. I know from me if it is working. All the days I spent in and out of psychiatric hospitals, sitting with psychologists, attending obesity clinics, diet clubs and knives and devices to cut me away, my answers for me were within me. All my days I wanted to read someone's story about compulsive overeating and wanted the recognition and understanding that someone else had lived through this. My story lay within me, buried underneath the flesh.

My life still throws s**t at me, like most people. I have money troubles, I have childcare problems, and I am involved in a legal matter with Abby's dad. I don't have an extended family for support and have a small circle of good friends, but my role, right now, is to take care of myself and my children. I feel privileged to be a mother and have gratitude to my body for allowing that to happen. I am confident that my children will grow up to be happy, balanced adults and I will do everything in my role to provide them with love, fun, joy, acceptance and childhood.

Me and men, well, I am still doing work with my counsellor on my relationships with men. I have to learn to trust and build up faith in men. But right at this point in my life, it is not a priority for me to be with anyone. I am enjoying getting to know me. I may also go back to college and get some of the education that I was robbed of in my childhood years. Now that my suffering and torture has been voiced, I feel it has now been put to bed. I realise that some things in life there won't be answers to or answers required. I also have the insight and understanding that life is here and now. The past is gone and the future is far away and I understand that the past took me to some scary places alongside the compulsion. Suffering from this compulsion, I don't know what the future holds, but it is not that important, it is the here and now that matters, getting to the end of the day and not have been in the pits of despair with food is recovery. I can't speak for tomorrow, but I can say no more surgery for me. It doesn't set the compulsion free. My head and heart require freedom and that's what my individual plan for me is all about and works for me. I hope I have never referred to myself in this book as F.A.T. As FAT for me will always be about my feelings and thoughts and each day I will learn to cope with my feelings and thoughts. Some days I sit and think, have I been a failure or success in this compulsion and I don't think there is any answer to that question, and I ask myself, would I use any of the methods of weight loss I have used in the past, and the answer to that, honestly, is no. I can answer that with complete honesty for the here and now. But I know how desperate I have become in the past, and I know what roads this cunning illness can take me down. But each second day, when I have to get the iron injections in my side and I look at the bruises on my body, I say enough is enough. This is one of the after effects of the stomach stapling; my body is not storing iron. I have had 3 blood transfusions and 7 months of iron injections into my hips. I also have investigations going on about my white blood cell count being so low and unable to fight infection. This may be another after effect of the stomach stapling…So no more for me. I feel I have done my sentence and, thankfully, I got underneath the flesh and found me and was able to realise that some answers and choices were deeply buried underneath what the knives tried to create a solution to.